A Palliative Ethic of Care

Clinical Wisdom at Life's End

Joseph J. Fins, MD

Chief, Division of Medical Ethics
Professor of Medicine
Professor of Public Health
Professor of Medicine in Psychiatry
Weill Medical College of Cornell University

Director of Medical Ethics
New York Presbyterian Hospital-Weill Cornell
Medical Center
New York, New York

JONES AND BARTLETT PUBLISHERS

Sudbury, Massachusetts

BOSTON   TORONTO   LONDON   SINGAPORE

World Headquarters

Jones and Bartlett Publishers
40 Tall Pine Drive
Sudbury, MA 01776
978-443-5000
info@jbpub.com
www.jbpub.com

Jones and Bartlett Publishers Canada
6339 Ormindale Way
Mississauga, Ontario L5V 1J2
CANADA

Jones and Bartlett Publishers International
Barb House, Barb Mews
London W6 7PA
UK

Jones and Bartlett's books and products are available through most bookstores and online booksellers. To contact Jones and Bartlett Publishers directly, call 800-832-0034, fax 978-443-8000, or visit our website, www.jbpub.com.

Substantial discounts on bulk quantities of Jones and Bartlett's publications are available to corporations, professional associations, and other qualified organizations. For details and specific discount information, contact the special sales department at Jones and Bartlett via the above contact information or send an email to specialsales@jbpub.com.

Library of Congress Cataloging-in-Publication Data
Fins, Joseph.
    A palliative ethic of care : clinical wisdom at life's end / Joseph Fins.
        p. ; cm.
    Includes index.
    ISBN 0-7637-3292-3 (alk. paper)
1. Palliative treatment. 2. Terminal care.
    [DNLM: 1. Terminal Care. 2. Advance Care Planning. 3.
Medical Futility. 4. Palliative Care. 5. Right to Die. WB
310 F516p 2005] I. Title.
    R726.8.F555 2005
    362.17′5—dc22

                                                                    2004030324

Production Credits
Executive Publisher: Christopher Davis
Production Director: Amy Rose
Editorial Assistant: Kathy Richardson
Associate Marketing Manager: Laura Kavigian
Manufacturing Buyer: Amy Bacus
Composition: Northeast Compositors
Text Design: Paw Print Media
Cover Design: Kristin E. Ohlin
Printing and Binding: Malloy, Inc.
Cover Printing: Malloy, Inc.

Printed in the United States of America
09 08 07 06 05   10 9 8 7 6 5 4 3 2 1

For Amy and Harry

Contents

Foreword

Over the last 15 years, the field of palliative care has grown exponentially. Increasing attention to the challenges and barriers that face this growing field of medicine are well articulated throughout this unique text. Palliative medicine is a young specialty defining its domain to improve the quality of living for those with serious illness; to take responsibility for managing patients' physical and psychological symptoms; and emphasizing a family-centered care model across multiple care systems.

To date, there are over 2000 physicians certified by the American Board of Hospice and Palliative Medicine and an application for subspecialty status has been submitted. More than 18 medical subspecialty professional organizations have signed on to a document that frames the Core Principle of Palliative Care. These organizations have committed themselves to educate their membership in the principles and practice of palliative care. Residency training programs are increasingly acknowledging the importance of trainees' competency in end-of-life care. Undergraduate and graduate medical education in palliative care is becoming more formalized with some physicians in training rotating on a palliative care inpatient unit or in a hospice program. Other trainees may only have some educational programs without an experiential elective.

A recent volume of *Academic Medicine* devoted most of its content to studies on the impact of a patient's death on physicians in training, identifying the critical need to support and mentor them through their patient's dying to reduce their significant distress

As well, a series of evidence based reports from the Institute of Medicine reviewing the current state of medical care of the dying in the United States identified healthcare professionals' lack of knowledge and education as a serious barrier to humane, compassionate care for patients and families.

This concise, two-part text takes up this educational imperative. It serves as a comprehensive primer on the ethics of end-of-life care starting with the ethical and legal principles essential to end-of-life decision making and ending with a practical methodologic approach and a pathway for clinical care.

Dr. Ned Cassem in his writings on the qualities necessary of a physician who cares for the dying identified the need for equanimity. This book models such equanimity by providing an understanding of the ethical principles that guide an approach to the seriously ill, possibly dying, patient and a way to translate them into goals of care.

The book's content has evolved from the author's rich and varied clinical experience in both ethics and palliative care. As the director for a clinical ethics consultation service in a tertiary academic medical center, Dr. Fins draws on his years of challenging case consultations that have often revolved around decision making at the end of life. The clinical issues are discussed in a way that provides an opportunity for physicians in training to learn how they might walk the last mile with their seriously ill patients as they negotiate life's final transition.

The book models how to doctor the dying. Specific attention is focused on the essential elements of ethical and palliative care consultations, communication, and symptom management with an emphasis on how to think about choosing an approach for an individual patient and family. By learning how to apply abstract ethical and legal principles to every day medical decision making, this uniquely relevant and readable text teaches students how to formulate a care plan that respects a patient's autonomy, dignity, and personhood. Dr. Fins developed the concept of a clinical pathway to operationalize and systematize end-of-life care, and his studies of the role of this assessment tool, the Goals of Care Assessment Tool, define its clinical usefulness as a practical approach to address the needs of patients and families who are trying to make difficult decisions in complex medical situations.

The book has a strong personal tone and quality that again reflects Dr. Fins's own process of learning how to care for this patient population. There is both a brilliance and a simplicity in the book's writing style. It is conversational and you feel as if you are on rounds with a master teacher. The complex decisions of deciding about the use of ventilators, about withholding and withdrawing care, or explaining brain death are addressed and you learn through the model conversations the words to say and the critical thinking necessary that starts with where the patient and family is and what they understand. Like making a medical diagnosis, you learn how to do a palliative care consultation—defining the problem, framing the issues, developing a strategy-consistent with a patient's goals for care and formulating a process that often begins with a patient and family meeting.

An important role for the book is to enhance physicians-in-training competency and level of comfort with talking about death and dying. Such death talk conversations are never easy but learning how to be sensitive, appropriate, and respectful is essential. Since physicians-in-training may not be exposed to role model clinicians educated in palliative care, the book provides an introduction to the field and sets a standard by which healthcare professionals should act.

Physicians-in-training who become knowledgeable about palliative care can use this text to advocate and challenge their physician teachers to prioritize the care of the dying to ensure competent and compassionate care for their patients.

Kathleen M. Foley, MD
Attending Neurologist
Pain & Palliative Care Service
Memorial Sloan-Kettering Cancer Center

Preface

The philosophy of this book was informed by my work as a medical ethicist at the intersection of ethical theory and everyday clinical practice. It is meant to be both theoretical and practical, informed by the view that the ability to effect real world change stems from deep knowledge of what we seek to reform. In this case, the object of reform is how we take care of patients and families at the end of life.

The relationship of ethical theory and clinical practice has long intrigued me. Since my days as a student interested in bioethics, it seemed to me that prevailing approaches to ethical questions in medicine and the life sciences were too deductive and prescriptive. Ethical principles seemed to exist in the abstract and were seemingly engrafted onto complex clinical scenarios without due concern for context. Although respect for ethical principles like autonomy, beneficence, nonmaleficence, and justice worked well in the seminar room, they seemed platitudinous and wanting at the bedside and in the clinic. While we all endorse these principles in theory, the challenge was to know which principle applied in practice given the unique clinical and narrative features of specific cases.

These questions led to the development of *clinical pragmatism*, a method of moral problem solving for clinical ethics and ethics case consultation.[1-5] Pragmatism as a school of thought seemed well-suited to address ethical questions in medical practice because of its interest in making a difference in the world and its embrace of uncertainty in human affairs. From the Greek *praxis*, pragmatism is about action—it's a philosophical method that seeks to link ideas with actions and actions with ideas. Theory informs practice and practical experience informs theory. It is a process of continual and evolving feedback, which builds on accruing knowledge. It is always aware of contingencies and our evolving understanding of the world.

Clinical pragmatism has its philosophical roots in the American pragmatic tradition of Oliver Wendell Holmes, Jr., William James, Charles Sanders Peirce, and the work of John Dewey in particular.[6-9] Dewey was the leading American philosopher of the first half of the twentieth century as well as a psychologist, democratic theorist, and educational reformer.[10-13] Deweyan pragmatism is an appealing philosophical method through which to view ethical challenges in clinical practice, and end-of-life care in particular.

Dewey had a real world perspective. He was interested in the intersection of theory and practice and had a strong interest in using the scientific method as a means to address normative questions.[14,15] His analytical approach was inductive. He drew heavily upon empirical observations to inform ethical reasoning about which principles should guide practice in a given case and lead to intelligent interventions.

But while principles matter in his pragmatism, Dewey was neither an essentialist nor a moral absolutist. Influenced by Darwin's work, he accepted the fact that advances in science and society called for an evolution in our thinking and mores. These advances were not to be feared or categorically proscribed, but rather understood as part of humankind's evolving history.

That Dewey accepted an evolving state of knowledge as normative makes his legacy especially relevant to the challenges, and opportunities, created at the end of life because of advances in life-sustaining therapies. Although his pragmatism would apply prevailing ethical principles to established or settled questions, he acknowledged that in novel circumstances one cannot know in advance which ethical principles matter or how competing principles might be balanced and specified.[16]

Building upon Dewey's pragmatism, clinical pragmatism sought to demonstrate that ethical principles were neither absolute nor fixed truths independent of context. Instead, principles are hypotheses that need to be understood and accepted in view of the consequence of their application in a particular narrative context.

In these ethically contingent cases, moral judgment is better served by a disciplined process of analysis, which attends to the facts and particulars under consideration. In this way, applicable principles can be delineated in order to discern consequent ethical responsibilities and obligations.

To help in the balancing and specification of principles, it is necessary to engage in a contextually situated analysis that Dewey called the process of *inquiry*. Inquiry is meant to be comprehensive and systematic. The objective is to consider all the material medical and narrative facts that would be necessary to make a reasonable judgment about a decision or course of action.

This process of inquiry is analogous to the inductive reasoning of differential diagnosis used in clinical medicine. And like that process of diagnosis, pragmatic inquiry begins with the recognition of what Dewey described as the *problematic situation*. A problematic situation is one that should prompt deeper reflection because ethical tensions are present but as yet unexplored or not fully appreciated.

Although brewing ethical problems may become obvious over time, the key is to identify them as early as possible so that an explicit process of inquiry may be brought to bear upon the problem. This is especially true with considering the ethical issues at the end of life. Inquiry can begin once the problematic situation has been made explicit.

When this occurs, it is possible to collect the medical, narrative, and contextual details necessary for the analytical process required to address the problem. This information leads to the articulation of an *ethics differential diagnosis*. These speculations in turn inform a negotiation with stakeholders about a plan of action, with the resultant consensus leading to an intervention. This process is completed with a periodic review that will foster experiential learning.

But too often, problems—like medical symptoms—are recognized too late in clinical practice and go unattended. Although these missed opportunities may become obvious in retrospect, they are often missed in real time. And with this, solvable problems morph into intractable dilemmas requiring the conflict-resolution skills of clinical ethicists and others.

Too often as a clinical ethicist, I have seen avoidable conflict turn into the sort of crisis that harms patients, divides families, and leaves clinicians stressed. Although ethics consultation can help to mediate many of these cases, the best ethics consult is one that never needs to be called. It is far better to identify brewing problems early on and intervene than to patch things up when things spin out of control.

The need to avoid these dilemmas and foster a "preventive ethic"[17] at the end of life led to the development of the Goals of Care Assessment Tool (GCAT).[18] The GCAT is a workable device structured to make the steps of pragmatic inquiry accessible to the practitioner. It is meant to have instrumental value, in the pragmatic tradition, and to help make a difference in the real world of patients and families. Step by step, the GCAT helps identify the sorts of triggers that represent a problematic situation that should prompt additional reflection and pragmatic inquiry, so that the care plan can best serve the goals of the patients and their families.

The GCAT builds upon clinical pragmatism and is pragmatic in its approach. But unlike clinical pragmatism, which was conceived for use by clinical ethicists, the GCAT was designed for clinicians. Though informed by ethical theory, it is accessible and practical.

The GCAT is also an educational prompt—a way of organizing knowledge to help students and trainees assemble the complex medical and narrative elements of a patient's case in a way that allows for meaningful intervention. Although we train our students and residents in physical diagnosis or how to examine a blood smear, we have not done a good job teaching them to systematically approach the care of patients throughout the life cycle, much less at the end of life. In this volume, the GCAT is used as an outline for instruction, providing the framework that links practical considerations about patient care with more theoretical concerns.

This mix of editorial objectives might strike some readers as discordant. Books like this one are generally thought to be either a workable text or a thoughtful mono-graph. It is expected that books in medicine or medical ethics are either theoretical or practical. To my mind this is an artificial and unproductive divide that impoverishes theory, practice, and patient care.

I have deliberately departed from such expectations and have sought to pragmatically blend both theory and practice. The book's first half is a theoretical and historical consideration about end-of-life care. The second half integrates theory and practice and seeks to provide practical wisdom, or *phronesis*, about the care of dying patients and their families.

I appreciate that seeking to write a book that is both a monograph on ethics and a textbook to educate and teach has the potential to confuse the reader. This is a risk worth taking. I believe that ethical theory and clinical practice are linked, and that the validation of theories about patient care is in medical practice itself. So instead of being jarred by its hybrid qualities, I hope that this little book will provide deeper insights into why end-of-life care is so challenging and how it can be improved.

My intention is to help foster needed reforms in how we die and I am confident that continued improvements are possible. Nonetheless, the tone of this book may seem pessimistic: that there is little to be done to improve the experience of dying patients and their families; that efforts at reform have had less than their hoped-for impact; and that patients lamentably remain at risk of overtreatment at the end of life. Sadly, that has been my take after a decade and a half of trying to make a difference in the way patients and families experience death and dying.

It is true that centers of excellence have sprung up to provide outstanding care, and that individual practitioners have developed first-rate training programs. Foundations have been generous with their support and this has helped to catalyze a cadre of practitioners who have begun to make palliative care a clinical discipline.

There is much to celebrate in improvements that have been made. But the reality remains that there still is a wide gap between what we teach and what gets done, and between rhetoric and deeds. Patients are still at risk if they have untreated pain or want to forgo aggressive curative therapies and opt for palliation. Although exemplary care will certainly be easier to achieve when the setting is conducive to its delivery, systemic reform, though necessary, is never sufficient to bring improvements to the care of individual patients and their families.

Although the GCAT could be an ingredient in systemic reform of clinical practice, we should be careful not to lose sight of the responsibility of individual practitioners for competent and compassionate care. The GCAT is designed to promote systemic reform by giving individuals the tools to both recognize patient needs and respond to them.

Whatever the system of care, the quality of its delivery hinges upon individuals, what he or she intuits and knows, and how each acts at the bedside. Ultimately, the delivery of care is provided by individuals who care: doctors prescribe pain medications; nurses administer them; chaplains console; and social workers work the bureaucracy to gain needed services. Each of us plays a part of a larger process, of course, but each of us needs to make our own singular contributions.

When all is said and done, the best palliative care that I have witnessed has been given when one individual has embraced the needs of another and become an advocate. It could be a courageous medical student who spoke up about the adequacy of pain relief, a nurse chiding a physician to accede to a patient's preferences, or a doctor quietly consoling a family after breaking bad news. These examples of *compassion*—from the French *to suffer with another*—are uniquely the acts of one individual for another. They are not systemic interventions. Systems of care are impersonal and anonymous. They do not suffer with the patient, though they can help shelter the efforts of dedicated practitioners. Although it may take a village to provide comprehensive palliative care in a complex institutional setting, it is the task of individual practitioners to initiate and sustain the provision of care. It is my hope that this volume will help them be better discerners of these systems of care so as to be better advocates for patients and their families.

I have written this book because I have faith in the individual practitioner—my colleagues in the helping professions. I believe that most of us came to clinical practice with idealism and a desire to make a difference in the world, if only we could be directed how to make compassion tangible. Although this book might be read as a critique of current practices, it is better understood as constructive criticism that will help translate good intentions into acts of kindness at life's end.

References

1   Fins JJ and Bacchetta MD. Framing the Physician-Assisted Suicide and Voluntary Active Euthanasia Debate: The Role of Deontology, Consequentialism, and Clinical Pragmatism. *Journal of the American Geriatrics Society* 43(5)(1995):563–568.

2   Fins JJ. From Indifference to Goodness. *Journal of Religion and Health* 35(3)(1996):245–254.

3 Fins JJ, Bacchetta MD, and Miller FG. Clinical Pragmatism: A Method of Moral Problem Solving. *Kennedy Institute of Ethics Journal* 7(2)(1997):129–145.

4 Fins JJ. Approximation and Negotiation: Clinical Pragmatism and Difference. *Cambridge Quarterly of Healthcare Ethics* 7(1)(1998):68–76.

5 Miller FG, Fletcher JC, and Fins JJ. Clinical Pragmatism: A Case Method of Moral Problem Solving. In *Introduction to Clinical Ethics*, 2nd ed. JC Fletcher, PA Lombardo, MF Marshall, and FG Miller, Frederick, (Eds.) Maryland: University Publishing Group, 1997.

6 Menand L. *The Metaphysical Club*. New York: Farrar, Straus and Giroux, 2001.

7 Dewey J. The Quest for Certainty. In *The Later Works*, Vol. 4: 1929. Carbondale: Southern Illinois University Press, 1988.

8 Dewey J. Theory of Valuation. In *The Later Works*, Vol. 13: 1938-1939. Carbondale: Southern Illinois University Press, 1991.

9 Dewey J. Logic: The Theory of Inquiry. In *The Later Works*, Vol. 12: 1938. Carbondale: Southern Illinois University Press, 1991.

10 Ryan A. *John Dewey and the High Tide of American Liberalism*. New York: W.W. Norton, 1995.

11 Hook S. *John Dewey: An Intellectual Portrait*. Amherst, New York: Prometheus Book, 1995.

12 Miller FG, Fins JJ, and Bacchetta MD. Clinical Pragmatism: John Dewey and Clinical Ethics. *The Journal of Contemporary Health Law and Policy* 13(27)(1996):27–51.

13 Fins JJ. Klinischer Pragmatismus und Ethik-Konsultation. (Clinical Pragmatism and Ethics Case Consultation). *Das Parlament* 49. Jahrgang/Nr. 23. 4 Juni 1999: p. 18.

14 Dewey J. *Experience and Nature*. Chicago and La Salle, Illinois: Open Court Publishing Company, 1997, pp. 134–137.

15 Dewey J. The Logic of Judgments of Practice. In *The Essential Dewey: Ethics, Logic, Psychology*. Vol 2. LA Hickman and TM Alexander, Eds. Bloomington: Indiana University Press, 1998, pp. 236–271.

16 Beauchamp TL and Childress JF. *Principles of Biomedical Ethics*. 4th ed. New York: Oxford University Press, 1994, pp. 28–37.

17 McCullough LB and Chervenak FA. *Ethics in Obstetrics and Gynecology*. New York: Oxford University Press, 1994.

18 Fins JJ, Miller FG, Acres CA et al. End-of-Life Decision Making in the Hospital: Current Practices and Future Prospects. *Journal of Pain and Symptom Management* 1999; 17(1):6–15.

Acknowledgments

This book would not have been possible without the lessons learned from the patients, families, and clinicians who have sought assistance from the Ethics Committee of New York Presbyterian Hospital—Weill Cornell Medical Center during the past decade. I am indebted to E. William Davis, Jr. for his vision in founding the committee and to Herbert Pardes and the late David B. Skinner for the honor of serving as its chair. Committee members have been a source of true collegiality and wonderful insights. I hope they will see some of their wisdom displayed in these pages.

Throughout this process I have been helped by many wonderful colleagues. Cathleen A. Acres was there at the beginning when we first envisioned goal setting as a way to structure end-of-life care and has made singular contributions to this volume throughout its writing. Franklin G. Miller, Matthew D. Bacchetta, and the late John C. Fletcher helped with the development of the philosophical framework that informs the pragmatic approach outlined here. Barbara Maltby added literary grace and a broader cultural perspective. Former Cornell medical students, Amy Kelley brought uncommon clinical sensibility to her review of the literature and provided useful insights into the trainee's perspective and Shantanu Agrawal added useful clinical material.

I am grateful to those who have read and commented on the book, especially David Kuhl for his close and insightful reading, Pablo Rodriguez del Pozo for reminding me that medical education can be transformative, and Ira Byock, Albert Jonsen, and Kathy Foley whose comments kindly grace this volume.

I am especially thankful for Dr. Foley's Foreword. I have been exceedingly lucky to have had her as a teacher and fortunate to have been able to participate in rounds on the Pain and Palliative Care Service at Memorial Sloan-Kettering Cancer Center while a Project on Death in America Faculty Scholar. Observing Dr. Foley and her colleague Russell Portenoy, now head of the Pain and Palliative Medicine Department at Beth Israel Medical Center in New York, was the ultimate exposure to excellence in palliative care.

Precisely because this book is written for students and trainees, I must acknowledge the many teachers and mentors who have taught me so much. First among them is the late John L. Battenfeld, a physician and humanist, whose practice remains worthy of emulation decades after his death. He exemplified the mix of compassion and technical competence to which the rest of us will long strive.

George B. Lieberman, Jeremiah A. Barondess, Morton D. Bogdonoff, Martin Gardy, Stanley Goldstein, and David E. Rogers have all been wise and wonderful mentors. I cannot imagine how different my life would have been had I not been guided by their wisdom and led by their example. In a similar vein I am indebted to Ralph Nachman, Alvin Mushlin, and Jack Barchas for encouraging me to pursue unconventional lines of scholarship and their unfailing support, administrative and otherwise. I appreciate their faith in me and hope that they will see the fruits of their confidence displayed here.

I am grateful to Antonio M. Gotto, Daniel Alonso, and Carol Storey-Johnson for the opportunity to develop new courses at Weill Medical College of Cornell University in clinical ethics and palliative care, which formed the basis of this text. I am particularly appreciative of the creative latitude they provided in curricular design and to the late David Clayson for his inspiring pedagogy. I have learned much from the many outstanding clinician-teachers who have taught so ably in our ethics and palliative care curriculum: Philip Lister, Kevin Kelly, Constance Peterson, Curtis Hart, Alan Gibofsky, Joseph T. Cooke, and David T. Mininberg.

Richard Cohen, C. Ronald MacKenzie, Anne Moore, Nicholas D. Schiff, H. Michael Ushay, David A. Silbersweig, Joseph T. Ruggiero, David H. Miller, James Clarke, Jeffrey D. Fisher, and Milton Viederman have all taught by example. I hope they see their own exemplary teaching efforts reflected in these pages.

To work at New York-Weill Cornell has been to be amongst a community of many dedicated professionals who rise to meet patient and family needs with idealism and compassion, some of whom are acknowledged here. Susan Mascitelli, Charles Miccoli, and their colleagues in Patient Services Administration have made our shared work in ethics consultation instructive and collaborative. Kathleen Burke has been a trusted advisor whose understanding of the intersection of the law and medicine is always humane and wise. William T. Greene, Steve Corwin, and Laura Forese have been steady supporters of our ethics program and fostered its growth. Anne Matier has made the impossible seem plausible, and often possible. I am also most appreciative of the daily support and dedication of Maureen Griffo.

I am also especially indebted to The Hastings Center, which remains an intellectual home away from home, and the many wonderful colleagues, past and present, who have made it such a special place: Daniel Callahan, Willard Gaylin, Strachan Donnelley, Tom Murray, James Nelson, Hilde Lindemann, Erik Parens, Bette Crigger, Ellen Moskowitz, Susan Wolf, Philip Boyle, Gregory Kaebnick, Erika Blacksher and Mark Hanson, and Bruce Jennings, who provided an opportunity to work on *Decisions Near the End of Life* and with Mildred Z. Solomon.

This work was funded, in part, by a grant from the Fan Fox and Leslie R. Samuels Foundation to explore the utility of goal setting in end-of-life care. I am most appreciative of their catalytic support of this project and generous underwriting of other activities in the Division of Medical Ethics, including research on the patient-proxy relationship.

Other foundations helped to underwrite research that informs this volume. I am grateful to have received a Project on Death in America Faculty Scholars Award to bridge the divide between clinical ethics and palliative care, the Woodrow Wilson National Fellowship Foundation for the opportunity to teach medical ethics on college campuses, and the Emily Davie and Joseph S. Kornfeld Foundation to develop clinical pragmatism as a method of moral problem solving. The United Hospital Fund Hospital Palliative Care Initiative underwrote research to delineate practice patterns at life's end and the Robert Wood Johnson Foundation provided a grant to Alan R. Fleischman and The New York Academy of Medicine for us to evaluate palliative care education in New York.

The Rev. and Mrs. John D. Twiname Remainder Trust funded collaborative efforts in pastoral care and the Committee on Campus Ministry of the Episcopal Diocese of New York supported ecumenical efforts to explore the interface of clinical ethics and religion. I am grateful to the Center for Learning and Leadership for supporting my collaboration with Daniel Brenner and Tsvi Blanchard. The Daniel and Janet Mordecai Foundation, the Wilson Bequest, and The Rosenstiel Foundation helped support our educational programs in medical ethics and end-of-life care.

I am especially grateful to Anne Coté Taylor for her enduring interest in our programs and her own pioneering work in patients rights, the Lucius N. Littauer Foundation, and the late Pamela Bromberg in particular, for support that led to the development of our initial educational programs at Cornell and the H.L. Bache Foundation for its partial support of work done at The Hastings Center. More recently, I have been supported by the Dana Foundation and the Buster Foundation to explore diagnostic and ethical issues related to disorders of consciousness.

I also would like to acknowledge the editorial support of Jones and Bartlett Publishers and Chris Davis, for his willingness to undertake this book, sound editorial advice, and enduring optimism. His accessibility and easy manner made writing this book possible even when I thought it would never be finished. I would also like to thank Amy Rose for all her efforts.

Finally, I want to acknowledge the love and support of my family. I wish my Mom were here so I could thank her for all her love and encouragement and the example of community service, which marked her all-too-brief life. Her legacy lives on in the work of my sister, Robin, who has been a trusted friend and advisor. I am glad that my dad got to read these pages and provided sagacious advice, that Harry saw them written from his high chair and babbled his comments, and that Amy and I can share this life and write its text together.

Joseph J. Fins

Permissions

The author gratefully acknowledges:

- Museu Picasso, Barcelona and The Picasso Administration, Paris for granting permission to reproduce Pablo Picasso's masterpiece *Ciencia y Caridad* on the cover. Copyright © (2005) Estate of Pablo Picasso/Artists Rights Society (ARS), New York.

The author acknowledges the courtesy of the following publishers for their kind permission to reproduce and excerpt from previously published work:

- The discussion on the culture of death and dying in America is excerpted and reprinted with permission from: Fins JJ, "Intimations of Reality and Immortality." *Generations: Journal of the American Society on Aging,* volume 23, issue 1, pages 81-86, published in 1999. Copyright © (1999) American Society on Aging, San Francisco, California. www.asaging.org

- The discussion on brain death objections is excerpted and reprinted with permission from: Fins JJ. "Approximation and Negotiation: Clinical Pragmatism and

Difference." *Cambridge Quarterly of Healthcare Ethics*, volume 7, issue 1, pages 68-76, published in 1998. Copyright © (1998) Cambridge University Press.

- The discussion of the origins of palliative care is excerped and reprinted with permission from: Fins JJ. "Principles in Palliative Care: An Overview." *Journal of Respiratory Care*, volume 45, issue 11, pages 1320-1330, published in 2000.

  Copyright © (2000) Daedalus Enterprises, Inc.

- The "Pain, Neuropsychologic, and Other Symptom" domains are reprinted with permission from: Meekin SA, Klein JE, Fleischman AR, and Fins JJ. "Development of a Palliative Education Assessment Tool for Medical Student Education."*Academic Medicine*, volume 75, issue 10, pages 986-992, published in 2000.

  Copyright © (2000) Lippincott Williams & Wilkins.

- The discussion on truth-telling and the origins of American bioethics is excerpted and reprinted with permission from: Fins JJ. Truth Telling and Reciprocity in the Doctor-Patient Relationship: A North American Perspective. In, *Topics in Palliative Care* Volume 5, pages 81-94. Bruera E and Portenoy RK, editors. New York: Oxford University Press, published in 2001.

  Copyright © (2001) Oxford University Press.

- An earlier version of the Goals of Care Assessment Tool (GCAT) appeared in, and is reprinted with permission from: Fins JJ, Miller FG, Acres CA, Bacchetta MD, Huzzard LL, and Rapkin BD. "End-of-Life Decision-Making in the Hospital: Current Practices and Future

Prospects." *Journal of Pain and Symptom Management*, volume 17, issue 1, pages 6-15, published in 1999.

About the Author

Joseph J. Fins, MD, FACP is Chief of the Division of Medical Ethics at Weill Medical College of Cornell University where he serves as Professor of Medicine, Professor of Public Health, and Professor of Medicine in Psychiatry. In addition, Dr. Fins is Director of Medical Ethics at New York-Presbyterian Weill Cornell Medical Center, Associate for Medicine at The Hastings Center, and a member of the Adjunct Faculty of Rockefeller University. He has been a Visiting Professor in Medical Ethics at The Complutense University in Madrid and is a recipient of a Soros Open Society Institute Project on Death in America Faculty Scholars Award, and a Woodrow Wilson National Fellowship Foundation Visiting Fellowship. In July 2000, Dr. Fins was appointed by President Clinton to the White House Commission on Complementary and Alternative Medicine Policy. A diplomat of the American Board of Internal Medicine, Dr. Fins is a graduate of Wesleyan University (BA with Departmental Honors, The College of Letters, 1982) and Cornell University Medical College (MD, 1986). He completed his residency in Internal Medicine and Fellowship in General Internal Medicine at The New York Hospital-Cornell Medical Center. Dr. Fins resides in Manhattan with his wife and son.

p a r t   I

Death and Dying in Context

c h a p t e r   o n e

Medical Students, Residents, and the Dying Patient

The physician's work lives on the confines of the shadow-land, and it might be expected that, if to any, to him would come glimpses that might make us less forlorn when in the bitterness of loss we cry . . .

—Sir William Osler[1]

The Challenge of Caring for the Dying

Caring for dying patients can be one of the most challenging—and potentially rewarding—responsibilities you will assume as a medical student or resident. These encounters can be professionally satisfying if done well and produce emotional distress if handled poorly. The odds are that you will not learn enough about the care of the dying in medical school and residency and that you will have to assume more

---

of a personal responsibility to develop necessary skills, knowledge, and expertise. This book is written to help you understand the needs of dying patients and their families and to give you deeper insights into why the provision of comprehensive end-of-life care remains a challenge for each of us as clinicians and for the health care system as a whole.

As a medical student or resident, when you meet dying patients you will also confront your own fear of dying. You will use defense mechanisms like denial that may distance you from the needs of your patients and foster what has been described as death avoidance. On rounds, this might be a decision to come back to see a dying patient who was sleeping later in the day. While this might appear to be a sympathetic approach to a patient who needs rest, closer examination of the team's motivations might reveal a discomfort of being around a patient who is cachectic, dyspneic, and clearly dying. Often times, the team does not return to see this dying patient and the task is left to the house officer or medical student who has been delegated this responsibility.

So you will return to this patient's bedside and gently wake him. You are uncertain if this is the right thing to do as he is sleeping and his sleep has been precious. Should a dying patient be examined when he is sleeping? Is that simply the routinization of care that we employ in hospitals? Is that good for this patient, or do I let him rest? You decide he needs to be awakened. After all you need to write your morning progress note. You reflect that "progress" in this context is a bit of an oxymoron. Progress to what? To death, to additional decline? These concerns haunt you even before you enter the patient's room.

You are now at the patient's bedside. He turns and sees you. He complains of shortness of breath and is slouched down in the bed. His lung exam is wet and he has rales two thirds up both lung fields. He is already on oxygen at a maximal setting and he has told you previously that he never wanted to be on a breathing machine. What can you do? Do you administer a diuretic by IV? Do you reexamine his preferences and offer the "comfort" provided by a ventilator? Do you write an order for some morphine to ease the work of breathing? Do you nebulize morphine? Or do you reposition him in bed and elevate his head?

If the patient were not dying, you believe that you would know what to do. But he is dying and you feel incompetent. Somehow the "full court press" does not make sense. He did not want that and you know in your heart that a stay in the intensive care unit will do little to prolong his life. It will just decrease the time his family can spend at his bedside, visiting hours in the unit such as they are. So you stand by at his side and think. No one has prepared me for this challenge. Yes, you know how to work up a pheochromocytoma, but what do you do for a dying guy with profound dyspnea?

As the patient looks at you imploringly for help, your spirits sink. You really don't know what to do, who to call for help, or where to begin. You start to question your competence. You realize that you haven't been trained to address questions of pain and symptom management at the end of life, much less talk with dying patients and their families about their needs and preferences. You ask yourself, where can I learn these technical skills and where can I acquire the judgment of the skilled physician caring for a dying patient? When does one know that enough is enough and less is perhaps more? These platitudes run through your mind and you begin to appreciate that they might just be platitudes for a good reason.

So where can you obtain these vital skills and clinical discernment? How do you gain this wisdom and insight? You have seen it on the wards, occasionally, maybe rarely. The engaged clinician, the communicator, who is technically skilled and humanistically oriented. He might be referred to as the medical school's "Osler," but you really don't want to be a semi-deity, you just want to be able to take care of dying patients and meet their needs.

Fortunately as you are ruminating about your ineptitude and comparing yourself to this physician–deity, an attending whom you do admire comes into the room. You are relieved that she has arrived and wipe the sweat that had been accumulating on your brow. You greet the attending and step aside, giving her the prime spot at the patient's bedside. This is an act of courtesy and respect, but you are also relieved that help has arrived. Your attending adjusts the patient's facemask and pillows and elevates the bed just a bit. She places her hand on the patient's shoulder and offers a comforting word. You don't quite hear what she says, but you can tell that the patient was consoled by the change in his expression. His breathing is as labored but the brow is now less furrowed. You watch and learn.

The doctor tells the patient that his shortness of breath can be controlled and that he will be comfortable. She reassures him that he will not have to go back to the ICU. "Don't worry," she says, again placing her hand on his shoulder. "We can manage all of this and keep you comfortable." All this time, time seemed to freeze and you wonder where she has found all the time for this. You rush around frantically trying to draw morning bloods, write your orders, and get through the day. But she sits at the patient's side with *aequanimitas*, a calmness that conveys to the patient that she has the time to meet his needs. You wonder how she does it.

Her solace is like a balm and you recall what you have heard about the therapeutic power of the doctor-patient relationship. You had always been a bit skeptical about this therapeutic power when you sat in lectures in the introduction to medicine course back in the first year of medical school, but now you are witnessing it first hand. With only a minor adjustment to his bed and a bit of tinkering with a facemask, this physician has brought comfort to this dying man. It could not be these technical adjustments that brought comfort but rather her presence in the room. Her confidence, her words, her engagement are what transformed discomfort into an eerie sort of ease.

As you watch, you ask yourself, how did she learn how to do this? You know you couldn't do what she just did, although you could have adjusted the bed and the facemask. She brought something more into the room. Was it simply the force of her personality? Or perhaps it was her superior knowledge that made the difference? Clearly, that does have something to do with her skill. But that is not all. She also probably benefited from effective mentoring and role models who taught her just as she might teach you. Her teachers helped her to develop both her scientific and humanistic skills in just the same way she is teaching you now, as you watch.

As you go through your training, you should seek out your own mentors. When you are lucky enough to find yourself in a situation like this, you should try to turn your frustration into a learning opportunity. But that is not enough. Seek out your own role models and mentors, doctors whom you admire, the ones to whom you might refer a loved one if they were in need of medical care. These *doctors' doctors* can teach you a lot about the art of doctoring, if you pay attention. As that sage Yogi Berra once said, "You can learn a lot by watching." And watch you should.

But unfortunately, not all stories of medical student or house staff frustration end as our fictional vignette. More often than not, you will be left in that room not knowing what to do with a patient in pain and distress. You might like to find a role model who will teach you, but you can't find one or are too shy to initiate a conversation. Sometimes, there will be a skilled practitioner who is ready to teach, but you are not yet ready to learn. At other times, you will be eager to learn and you will be surrounded by attendings who seem exclusively focused on curing, having forgotten the art of caring.

Despite these challenges—those within yourself and those within your institution—you still must learn how to care for dying patients and their families. You owe it to them and you owe it to yourself to develop these skills. Patients and families will expect this of you and it is your ethical obligation to meet this responsibility.

I have written this book to help you fulfill these obligations. It is both a practical guide to thinking about caring for patients at the end of life and a way to explore your own thoughts about your growing professionalism. Other books will focus more comprehensively on the technical aspects of end-of-life care such as drug dosing or the management of common symptomatology. This volume will do some of that but the goal is a bit more ambitious. It is to teach you how to make *judgments* about patient care at life's end and help you develop the clinical discernment that seems so difficult to obtain and which you so admire in the skilled physician.

Though this book is not a substitute for rounds with a skilled and compassionate clinician, it can be thought of as a virtual rounds and give you opportunities to think through common and challenging clinical scenarios at the end of life by offering a conceptual approach to help you analyze new and novel situations.

Goal-Setting Near the End of Life

This conceptual approach centers around the framework of *goal-setting*. Simply put, if we can determine what the goals of the patient and family are, then we can set out to meet them. In real life, this means overcoming the routinization of care decisions that often lead to an escalation of care when this was neither desired nor likely to influence the outcome. If we were to invoke a soundbite, it might be: instead of letting available technology drive the goals of care, let the goals of care drive the therapy.

This may seem a bit simplistic or platitudinous but our experience has shown that the articulation of the goals of care can provide valuable guidance in directing care at the end of life, especially when there are conflicting perspectives about the "right thing to do." This methodology has grown out of our work in ethics case consultation at a large academic medical center, empirical research on end-of-life practice patterns, and the teaching of medical students and residents. In each of these activities, and our own work as clinicians caring for dying patients and their families, we have found that simply asking about what the goals of care are can help clarify preferences and clinical priorities.

I have seen this most clearly from my work in ethics case consultation in which most conflicts at the end of life emanated from discordance between goals of care. Most of the time these conflicts were not because of a principled ethical difference about a proper course of action but rather from a failure to communicate and get everyone on the same page. When my colleagues and I facilitate discussions—between patients, families, and the clinical team—we have been able to achieve a consensus in upwards of 75% of cases that were brought to our ethics committee using goal setting as an organizing principle.

From these clinical activities and our research in the sociology of death and dying in the acute care setting, we have developed a structured method of goal setting that you will be able to use in your own work as clinicians. The centerpiece of this method is the Goals of Care Assessment Tool or GCAT. We will discuss the GCAT in detail in this volume, and apply it to paradigmatic cases, to help you learn how to better assess the needs of patients and families near the end of life as your clinical responsibilities grow.

How This Book Is Organized

In addition to describing the practical uses of the GCAT and applying it to challenging cases, we will also discuss the context within which you will be trying to provide better end-of-life care. In these efforts, I have kept in mind that cases can look very different when seen from the vantage point of a medical student or resident. Inexperience and medical hierarchies can alter perceptions and confound decision making. So I have tried to write a book that remains cognizant of your stage of training and of your needs and unique concerns. I have attempted to see cases from your point of view and appreciate the challenges encountered when you are not the attending and not in charge.

To meet the needs of the busy student or resident, the book is divided into two parts, which can be used as stand-alone modules, if you choose. Part I is a review of the history of palliative care and modern bioethics and considers how these two movements have influenced our thinking about the needs of patients at the end of life. We will then turn to how this history informed legal practices governing the care of the dying. We will consider pertinent legal issues such as informed consent and refusal and decisions to forgo life-sustaining therapies through do-not-resuscitate orders and advance directives. This grounding in the law will allow us to understand current end-of-life practice patterns in the modern American hospital and how and when these critical decisions are undertaken.

With this background, Part II provides a detailed clinical strategy (designed specifically for medical students and residents) to enable you to identify the goals of care for patients near the end of life. The GCAT will be introduced as a communication tool in demonstrating the importance of clear and competent communication when dealing with the sensitive issues that come up at life's end. I will describe ways to develop good communication skills, while also discussing common causes of miscommunication that complicate end-of-life care. Most critically you will learn how the GCAT can help you organize care and orchestrate effective communication *when cure is no longer the prevailing goal of care*. This framework is enriched with examples drawn from clinical experience.

Closing Words

When you arrived at medical school you probably had idealistic goals. I hope that this volume will help you reaffirm those aspirations and give you the tools to relieve pain and suffering at the end of life, the courage to be a humane and concerned physician, and the appreciation of palliative care as a gift you can give to your patients. I also hope that this book will help you better appreciate your ethical obligation to develop the competence to provide this care.

Most importantly, I hope that you will have the courage to be an advocate for the comprehensive care of the dying even if that means going against the grain. If you step up to the plate, you won't change the world but you will have a positive impact on your patients and their families and ultimately your own students. One day they will look to you as a role model of exemplary practice at the end of life.

Reference

1 Osler W. *Science and Immortality.* Boston and New York: Houghton, Mifflin & Co, 1904.

c h a p t e r   t w o

The Rise of Bioethics and Palliative Care Movements

Why is palliative care so difficult to do? Why does every hospital have an intensive care unit while few have a palliative care service or unit designated for the care of the dying? Why do medical schools give scant attention to end-of-life care? Don't we all share this common thread of mortality? Won't we all die? You will graduate from medical school and be able to prescribe antibiotics but many residents remain uncomfortable with the provision of pain medications. Why is this the case?

To put these challenges into context so that you might better understand the clinical world that will harbor your practice, we need to consider societal attitudes to death and dying. To do this we will review the origins of palliative care and the interplay between that social movement, patients' rights, and bioethics.

We will review the development of palliative care in the United States and in Europe, most notably in Great Britain, and see that each has distinct philosophical roots and antecedents. This history continues to inform the challenges that you will confront when you advocate for better end-of-life care. As we will see, palliative care in Great Britain grew out of a religious tradition and concerns about social solidarity. The nascent American palliative care movement, in contrast, gained prominence in response to secular and legal developments that began with the assertion of patients' rights in the 1960s and culminated in the debate over physician-assisted suicide in the 1990s.

The relationship between physician-assisted suicide and palliative care in American medicine remains complicated. Although palliative care should be judged on its own merits, it is often seen through the prism of an ideological stance about physician-assisted suicide.[1]

European Origins of Hospice and Palliative Care

To help bring palliative care principles to the bedside, we first need to understand their origins.[2] Palliative care has its origins in the hospice movement—a word that derives its meaning from two Latin roots: *hospis*, which means both host and guest, as well as *hospitium*, the venue where hospitality was given and received. Most commentators would maintain that the modern development of hospice was started in Great Britain by Dame Cicely Saunders. Dame Cicely founded the world's most famous hospice, St. Christopher's Hospice outside of London.[3]

Palliative care has deep religious roots. Dame Cicely has explicitly acknowledged the theological foundation of her life's work. Commenting on the religious affiliations of her colleagues at St. Christopher's she observed that, "We are not all Christians here, by any means, but our work is done in the obedience to the Christian imperative. For me personally, it could not be done otherwise."[4] Some commentators have viewed the spiritual roots of hospice care as a reaction to the technological coldness of modern medical practice and the need to find meaning in death and dying and human finitude. The distinguished historian of medicine Roy Porter has observed, " . . . that, given scientific medicine's inability to give any meaning, and maybe any dignity, to dying, the hospice movement has arisen, as an essentially Christian framework to cope with our going out."[5]

While we would maintain that good end-of-life care need not be motivated by a religious orientation—and is itself a secular good—it is important to acknowledge the religious origins of palliative care. Dame Cicely appreciated these important roots and, in her own scholarly writings, has traced the hospice movement to Fabiola, the Fourth century Roman matron and disciple of St. Jerome who offered food, drink, shelter, clothing, and lodging to needy strangers.

This tradition was continued within monastic hospices into the Middle Ages where pilgrims and other travelers found assistance and care. Pilgrims would trek to shrines such as those in Rome, Jerusalem, or Santiago de Compostela in Spain and stay at refuges or shelters en route. Many of these pilgrims were sick and seeking a cure at their destinations and died along the way in these hospices.

The special link between hospice work and the care of the dying dates to the 19th Century. In 1842 Mme. Jeanne Garnier opened a hospice for dying cancer patients in Lyons. In 1879 Our Lady's Hospice in Dublin was opened by the Irish Sisters of Charity whose primary focus was explicitly on the care of the dying.[6] It has been reported that the Sisters said, "It is not a hospital, for no one comes here expecting to be cured. Nor is it a home for incurables, as the patients do not look forward to spending years in the place. It is simply a 'hospice' where those who are received have very soon to die, and who know not where to lay their weary heads."[7]

The founder of the Irish Sisters of Charity, Mother Mary Aikenhead, brought her order to England in 1905 to found St. Joseph's Hospice. Around the same time a physician, Dr. Howard Barrett, founded St. Luke's Home for the Dying Poor in 1893. Barrett, somewhat lost to history, is an important figure in the evolution of palliative medicine because he pioneered the regular use of morphine *around the clock* so as to minimize patient distress.

Cicely Saunders began her own training at St. Luke's in 1948 when she arrived as a twenty-nine-year-old social worker with a nursing degree. Following the unheralded lead of Barrett's work with morphine at St. Luke's, Saunders began her own pioneering work in opioid clinical pharmacology and pain management. When she moved on to St. Joseph's Hospice in 1958—after going to medical school in her late thirties—she broadened her work on pain management to include the psychosocial dimensions of death, dying, and bereavement. In 1967 she founded St. Christopher's Hospice and her charismatic leadership is credited with launching the modern palliative care movement.[2]

These efforts coalesced in 1990 when the World Health Organization (WHO) convened an Expert Committee to disseminate the message of pain control and palliative care to an international audience. This group also articulated the modern definition of palliative care as ". . . the active total care of patients whose disease is not responsive to curative treatment. Control of pain, of other symptoms, and of psychological, social, and spiritual support is paramount. The goal of palliative care is the achievement of the best quality of life for patients and their families."[8] This definition highlights the importance of symptom management over cure and asserts a mandate for comprehensive care. It is more than the absence of certain curative interventions and is an important articulation of the practitioner's affirmative obligations to dying patients and their families.[9,10] This broadens the unit of care and suggests that palliative medicine transcends the traditional boundaries of the doctor-patient dyad, both by including the needs of families and by addressing psychosocial and spiritual needs in addition to clinical ones.

The American Context

It is notable as we recount this history to observe that, thus far, we have spoken of international developments in palliative care and not work done in the United States. This is because the palliative care movement was slow to develop in America. European-born, Dr. Elisabeth Kübler-Ross first pierced "long-held taboos on discussing and studying death" in the 1960s while teaching at the University of Chicago Medical School[11] and with the publication of "On Death and Dying" in 1969.[12] Nonetheless, the cultural transformation that she helped to catalyze was difficult to effect. The first hospice was founded in Connecticut under the leadership of former Health, Education, and Welfare Secretary, Joseph Califano in 1974 and palliative care has been slow to take root.[13] This reflects differing cultural norms between American and European medicine that continue to inform medical practice.

Commentators have distinguished European and American medicine in a number of fundamental ways that have a bearing on care at the end of life. The predominant ethical principles governing European healthcare are justice and social solidarity. Everyone is assured access to care, even if one's choice of care is constrained or limited. In the United States, these concerns about distributive justice have been subsumed by the premium we have placed on self-determination. At the risk of simplification, this has led not to a right to care but to a right to make the choice to refuse life-sustaining therapies.

This difference can be explained in part by the principles that motivated American medical ethics during this time. In contrast to the European experience, American medical ethics stressed the promotion of patient autonomy and asserted the negative right to be left alone. The American focus has been on the promulgation of legal protections that would allow care to be withheld or withdrawn and the exercise of choice.[14] The motivation for changing how we die was not a religious one but a means to resist the seductive technological imperative that marks American medicine.[15] Central in this was the importance of choice and the information that one needs to make informed choices. Self-determination, not the communitarian ethic that informed palliative care in Europe, was what guided the evolution of practice in the United States. As the palliative care movement took root in Europe, a bioethics movement focusing on the rights of patients to exercise choice grew in the United States, embracing an autonomy ethic far more expansive than our colleagues around the world.[16]

Because of these forces, the hospice and palliative care movement, which was becoming integrated into the continuum of care abroad, remained marginalized in America. The WHO plea for "the active total care of patients whose disease is not responsive to curative treatment" was discordant in an era obsessed by either the promise or the peril of medical technology. In this context, an attempt to employ technology in the service of pain and symptom management was difficult to realize in the medical mainstream. For these reasons, hospice emerged as a set of services that were delivered outside of the hospital setting and within local communities. The American hospice—in contrast to its European counterpart—was outside the medical mainstream and a reaction to its excesses, notably the overuse of medical technology.

The Rise of Self-Determination

American practice patterns began to break from tradition in 1914 when the great jurist Benjamin Cardozo articulated the right of adult competent patients to consent to treatments.[17] Writing while still a judge on the New York State Court of Appeals in *Schloendorff vs. the Society of The New York Hospital*, Cardozo opined that "Every human being of adult years in sound mind has a right to determine what shall be done with his own body; and a surgeon who performs an operation without the patient's consent commits an assault for which he is liable for damages . . . This is true except in cases of emergency when the patient is unconscious and when it is necessary to operate before consent can be obtained."[18]

Although this articulation of informed consent rings true to the modern reader, Cardozo's opinion was a departure from historical norms. Throughout the history of medicine, palliation and truth telling have been at odds. If palliation was seen as a way to preserve hope, then the truth was the enemy of hope and frequently hidden from the patient's view. Palliation was not about disclosure but as its 17th Century usage suggests, cloaking or disguising the truth.[19] Traditionally, as the psychiatrist and legal scholar Jay Katz has observed, the doctor-patient relationship was silent when it came to sharing the truth.[20]

While today we may embrace a more expansive view of palliative care that requires patients to know their circumstances and the truth about their diagnosis and prognosis, until very recently patients were felt to be served by less, not more information—especially when the news was bad and there was little to offer. Indeed, if we are honest with ourselves, we must admit that our clinical intuitions tell us that sharing a grave diagnosis with a patient has to be antithetical to the promotion of palliation. If the goals of palliation are to relieve pain, minimize suffering, and protect vulnerable patients from unnecessary burdens, it would seem unlikely that the truth could be comforting.

But a deeper examination of this stance suggests that patients do in fact have the right to know the truth about their conditions in order to make choices and live fully. Self-reflection and authentic encounters with loved ones can not be accomplished through a veil of deception. A dying patient can not find meaning in the dying process if he does not know he is dying. Indeed if we value meaning, we must also value the truth. Understood this way the truth is not the enemy of hope, but is itself a palliative and a comfort.

This line of reasoning, so central to modern notions of informed consent and patient self-determination, has its origins in Cardozo's decision, although the significance of his decision was not appreciated at the time. Even twenty-five years after the decision, legal scholars commemorating Cardozo's legacy did not even mention this informed consent opinion in a memorial law review volume jointly sponsored by the Harvard, Columbia, and Yale Law schools.[21] Although this 1939 collection cited *Schloendorff*, it cited an aspect of the opinion that was unrelated to informed consent and asserted a malpractice exemption for hospitals that provided charity care. It should come as no surprise that this aspect of *Schloendorff* has been overruled and that today we remember this decision for its prescience notion of informed consent.

A 1949 text on legal medicine did cite *Schloendorff* but it only gave lip service to informed consent. Even at that juncture, the author L. J. Regan advocates a more traditional and paternalistic model of the doctor-patient relationship. Commenting on consent prior to surgery, he counsels readers to envision the relationship between physician and patient as, ". . . one of trust and confidence. It is submitted that the best interest of the patient is served in trusting his welfare to the skill and integrity of the physician." [22] This view was typical of medical practice patterns through the 1950s, although some early empirical studies suggested that some cancer patients were beginning to express a desire to know their diagnosis.[23]

While these views foreshadowed changes in clinical practice that would take place within a decade, the prevailing medical ethic of this period remained paternalistic. This is captured in Oken's often-cited study of physicians at Michael Reese Hospital published in 1961.[24] Oken observed that 90% of physicians reported they withheld the diagnosis when their patients had cancer. When information was shared, disclosure was limited or deliberately misleading in order to ". . . sustain and bolster the patient's hope." Although earlier patient surveys demonstrated that patients wanted to know their diagnosis, Oken observed that physicians he studied disagreed. He wrote that, "The vast majority of these doctors feel that almost all patients really do not want to know, *regardless of what people say*. [italics added] They approach the issue with the view that disclosure should be avoided unless there are positive indications, rather than the reverse."

Toward an Ethic of Patients' Rights

Paternalistic attitudes toward truth telling and the patient's right to know his or her diagnosis began to change dramatically in the years following Oken's study.[25] When Oken's inquiry into physician attitudes toward truth telling was repeated by Novack and colleagues in 1979, a full 97% of practitioners ". . . indicated a preference for telling a cancer patient his diagnosis." The authors characterized this change as a "complete reversal of attitude" since Oken made his observations.[26]

Tracing the evolution of practice patterns is a far easier task than attempting to explain why these changes occurred. Some have maintained that disclosure of the truth was made easier by improvements in treatment. When the truth was not directly equated with the erosion of all hope, it became easier to be forthcoming.[27]

Although technological advances surely played a role in these changes, the emergence of truth telling in medical practice was influenced more by factors outside of medicine. In many respects, the decline of physician paternalism was a broader reflection of the times and the social turbulence that convulsed the nation in the 1960s. These forces, external to medicine, reconfigured all aspects of American life and influenced how physicians and patients communicated with each other. The emergence of assorted "rights movements" asserting the rights of minorities, women, and consumers inevitably led to a broader articulation of patient's rights. If citizens enjoyed new rights in civil life, and consumers had increased protections in the market place, then patients were also logically entitled to know about their medical condition if they became ill.

America's preoccupation with rights in the 1960s also led to the birth of modern medical ethics. Like other rights movements of that era, medical ethics sought to minimize hierarchies and promote the individual's self-determination. More importantly, in illustrating the possibilities of patient self-determination, medical ethics demonstrated the limitations of physician paternalism.

The emerging field of medical ethics suggested that some clinical decisions were more than technical determinations: they were *value choices* that drew upon a patient's beliefs and mores. Because these values were highly personal—and at times idiosyncratic—the patient was best positioned to make these decisions. However well-intentioned a physician might be, he could not decide what was in the patient's best interest or what counted as "good."[28] These decisions were outside the purview of the physician's expertise and thus the inappropriate object of paternalism. Patients had to make these judgments for themselves and be given the necessary information they would need to make these decisions. Simply put, patients would need to know the truth. For, as Edmund Pellegrino has noted, the ". . . human capability for autonomous choices cannot function if truth is withheld, falsified, or otherwise manipulated."[29]

Structural changes in the delivery of care during this period also fostered this emerging autonomy ethic. During the 1960s medical care became more impersonal and anonymous. The dyadic doctor-patient relationship was increasingly replaced by more complex care arrangements, especially when the patient was near death. The local physician who made house calls and took care of the entire family's medical needs was replaced by a team of doctors working in offices and clinics outside the neighborhood. The rise of medical technology, coupled with the restructuring of health care financing, moved care from the home to the hospital. Care became increasingly institutionalized.

Gone were the days of the general practitioner who delivered your parents and took care of your ear infections when you were in grade school. He was replaced by specialists of all stripes and overall patient care became more fragmented.

As the general practitioner was replaced by a new generation of doctors, the GP's style of doctor-patient communication also went out of fashion. The guidance that once seemed appropriate and sensitive from a trusted neighborhood physician was increasingly perceived as too directive when it came from a virtual stranger who did not know you, much less your parents or grandparents. Advice that was once appreciated from one source seemed to be an intrusion when it came from another. Such counsel was soon labeled pejoratively as paternalistic; and it probably was.

These physicians did not know their patients as their predecessors in general practice did. When this younger generation of physicians tried to use their own values as a proxy for their patients, it became increasingly clear that doctor and patient now inhabited different worlds. With the fragmentation of care, the broader institutionalization of medical practice, and the rapid escalation of physician incomes beginning in the 1960s, physician and patient were less likely to hail from the same cultural background, pray in the same congregation, or share the same socioeconomic class. This social dislocation made old style paternalism increasingly untenable, if not impossible.

In this emergent environment, the patient's voice had to be heard. Physicians who did not know their patients could not speak for them and if the physician could no longer speak for their patients, patients had to speak for themselves and exert their self-determination and autonomous choice.

But patient self-determination became more than a vehicle for self-expression. It soon became a protection against vestigial paternalism and a defense against the beliefs, values, or prejudices of the practitioner. This became especially important when people of different cultural and faith traditions began to come together to provide and receive health care. Although this diversity enriches America's cultural life, this same diversity can create challenges when moral dilemmas arise in the practice of medicine.

Unlike other nations with a dominant religion, we do not have a single religious tradition to turn to for guidance. Instead, we have a plurality of traditions capable of responding to ethical dilemmas in patient care. A secular ethic, with its emphasis on patient autonomy was especially well-suited to the American context in contrast with the European palliative care movement which, as we have seen, drew heavily upon Christian theology for inspiration.

Stressing patient self-determination as its overriding principle, secular bioethics laid the ground rules for adjudicating moral dilemmas in patient care when cultural mores clash. Tolerance would prevail and the patient's values would have primacy. Although the stakeholders would not necessarily have to agree with the patient's beliefs, all would accept the importance of pluralism and accommodation. In a complicated world, secular bioethics allowed a diversity of peoples to pursue their beliefs and be "different without being deviant."[30] It did not necessarily promote the provision of comprehensive palliative care, but it did allow patients

greater opportunities to refuse life-sustaining medical therapies. As we will see, this was a necessary but still an insuffi-
cient advance on the road to improved end-of-life care in
America.[31]

References

1 Fins JJ and Bacchetta MD. Framing the Physician-Assisted Suicide and
Voluntary Active Euthanasia Debate: The Role of Deontology, Consequentialism, and Clinical Pragmatism. *Journal of the American Geriatrics Society* 43(5)(1995):563–568.

2 This discussion of the origins of palliative care is based upon and contains excerpts from: Fins JJ. Principles in Palliative Care: An Overview.
Journal of Respiratory Care 45(11)(2000):1320–1330.

3 du Boulay S. *Cicely Saunders: Founder of the Modern Hospice Movement.* London: Hodder and Stoughton, 1984.

4 James N and Field D. The Routinization of Hospice: Charisma and
Bureaucratization. *Social Science & Medicine.* 34(12)(1992):1363–
1375.

5 Porter R. Religion and Medicine. In *Companion Encyclopedia of the History of Medicine.* WF Bynum and R Porter, Eds. New York: Routledge,
1997, p. 1465.

6 Saunders C. The Evolution of Hospices. *Free Inquiry.* (Winter
1991/92): pp. 19–23.

7 Goldin G. *Work of Mercy.* Ontario, Canada: Associated Medical Services and The Boston Mills Press, 1994, p. 270.

8 World Health Organization. *Cancer Pain Relief and Palliative Care.*
Geneva, Switzerland: World Health Organization, 1990, pp. 11–12.

9 Working Party on Specialist Palliative Care (J Wiles). Specialist Pallia-
tive Care: A Statement of Definitions. Occasional Paper 8. London:
National Council of Hospice and Specialist Palliative Care Services,
October 1995.

10 Meier DE, Morrison RS, and Cassel CK. Improving Palliative Care.
Annals of Internal Medicine 127(3)(1997):225–30.

11 Noble HB. Elisabeth Kübler-Ross, 78, Dies; Psychiatrist Revolutionized
the Care of the Terminally Ill. *The New York Times.* August 26, 2004,
p. B-8.

12 Kübler-Ross E. *On Death and Dying.* New York: Touchstone, 1997.

13 Califano, Claudia. Personal Communication.

14 President's Commission for the Study of Ethical Problems in Medicine and Biomedical and Behavioral Research. *Deciding to Forego Life-Sustaining Therapy.* Washington, DC: US Government Printing Office, 1983.

15 Callahan D. *The Troubled Dream of Life: Living with Mortality.* New York: Simon and Schuster, 1993.

16 Surbone A. Truth Telling to the Patient. *Journal of the American Medical Association* 268(1992): 1661–1662.

17 This discussion on truth-telling and the origins of American bioethics is based upon and contains excerpts from: Fins JJ. Truth Telling and Reciprocity in the Doctor-Patient Relationship: A North American Perspective. In *Topics in Palliative Care* Vol. 5. Bruera E and Portenoy RK, Eds. New York: Oxford University Press, 2001, pp. 81–94.

18 *Schloendorff v Society of New York Hosp,* 211 N.Y. 125 (1914).

19 Fins JJ. Palliation in the Age of Chronic Disease. *The Hastings Center Report* 22(1)(1992):41–42. Reprinted in *Cases in Bioethics: Selections from the Hastings Center Report,* 2nd Ed.. New York: St. Martin's Press, 1993.

20 Katz J. *The Silent World of Doctor and Patient.* New York: The Free Press, 1984.

21 Essays dedicated to Mr. Justice Cardozo. *Columbia Law Review* vol. XXXIX, no. 1; *Harvard Law Review* LII, no. 3; *Yale Law Journal* XLVIII, no. 3. January 1939.

22 Regan LJ. *Doctor and Patient and the Law.* 2nd ed. St. Louis: The C.V. Mosby Company, 1949.

23 Kelly WD and Friesen SR. Do Cancer Patients Want To Be Told?" *Surgery* 27(6)(1950):822–826.

24 Oken D. What to Tell Cancer Patients. *Journal of the American Medical Association* 175(1961):1120–1128.

25 Klenow DJ and Youngs GA. Changes in Doctor/Patient Communication of a Terminal Prognosis: A Selective Review and Critique. *Death Studies* 11(4)(1987):263–277.

26 Novack DH, Plummer R, Smith RL, et al. Changes in Physicians' Attitudes Toward Telling the Cancer Patient. *Journal of the American Medical Association* 241(1979):897–900.

27 Pentz R. Hope. Presented at the Eighth Annual Bioethics Summer Retreat. Copper Mountain Resort, Colorado, June 21, 1996.

28 Veatch RM. Why Physicians Cannot Determine if Care is Futile. *Journal of the American Geriatrics Society* 42(1994):871–874.

29 Pellegrino ED. Is Truth Telling to the Patient a Cultural Artifact? *Journal of the American Medical Association* 268(1992):1734–1735.

30 Fins JJ. Encountering Diversity: Medical Ethics and Pluralism. *The Journal of Religion and Health* 33(1)(1994):23–27.

31 Fins JJ, Peres J, Schumacher JD, and Meier C. *On the Road from Theory to Practice: Progressing Towards Seamless Palliative Care.* Washington, DC: Last Acts National Program Office, Robert Wood Johnson Foundation, 2003.

c h a p t e r   t h r e e

Death, Dying, and the Law

The Law and the Rise of Patient Self-Determination

A consideration of the forces that advanced truth telling and, ultimately, patient self-determination in North American medicine would be incomplete without acknowledging the important role played by the law during this period.[1] Broader social changes, like the emergent rights movements of the 1960s, were able to infiltrate the sequestered world of medical practice through the growing influence of the courts. Judicial activity during this period dramatically altered the clinical landscape with decisions advancing the centrality of informed consent and patient autonomy. Indeed, it would not be an exaggeration to suggest that the legal system became the vector by which the old paternalism was breached and replaced by a new strain of patient self-determination.

Patient self-determination was promoted through a new genus of informed consent cases, which considered both the patient's right to medical information and his/her place in medical decision-making. Early cases from this period hinged upon questions of disclosure—what the patient would need to know to make an informed decision about his/her care.[2,3] These cases first articulated the physician's affirmative obligation to share important information with the patient.[4] Subsequent cases specified what constituted *reasonable* disclosure about a patient's illness and treatment options.[5-7] More stringent requirements for disclosure naturally led to greater patient involvement in medical decision making. And as patients became more knowledgeable about their circumstances they came to expect a greater role in medical decision making.

Quinlan and the Right to Die

End-of-life care was a central area in which patients and families wanted to have greater say in decision making. This negative right to be left alone, to die, was first established in patients with overwhelming cognitive impairment like the persistent vegetative state.[8] In this context, the withdrawal of life-sustaining therapy was more justifiable because of the gravity of the patient's condition and the lack of any efficacious treatment.[9] An important case in the evolution of a right to die was that of Karen Ann Quinlan in 1976.[10] Quinlan was a high school student when she lapsed into permanent unconsciousness. Her family petitioned the court for her ventilator to be removed and the New Jersey Supreme Court granted their request.[11]

The court honored the request of her parents to remove the ventilator in large part because of the futility of any further interventions. She had been diagnosed as being in a persistent vegetative state, a state of permanent unconsciousness, described by B. Jennett and F. Plum in 1972.[12,13] Based on Dr. Plum's personal examination of Ms. Quinlan[14] and the gravity of her condition, the court justified the removal of life support. They asserted that such an action was ethically appropriate because she was hopelessly unconscious and had lost the possibility of ever returning to a "cognitive sapient state."[15] Her ventilator was removed but she continued to breathe because her brain stem was intact. Supported by excellent nursing care and artificial nutrition and hydration, she survived for years.

While the emerging right to die began in those with overwhelming brain injury, this right to self-determination gradually became progressively more expansive. Increasingly, society saw these as highly personal choices and not merely technical ones determined by one's diagnosis and prognosis under the purview of the doctor alone. Individuals had the right to refuse therapy and to withdraw their consent for continued life-sustaining interventions in the name of self-determination.

The societal consensus to direct one's care, even if a decision might result in one's death, developed in the wake of the Quinlan case. It became ensconced in the 1983 report written by the President's Commission for the Study of Ethical Problems in Medicine and Biomedical and Behavioral Research. Appropriately entitled, *Deciding to Forego Life–Sustaining Treatment*, the President's Commission report laid out ethical justifications for the refusal of unwanted medical interventions and became the basis for state laws that allow for natural death and orders to forgo resuscitation through do-not-resuscitate (DNR) orders.[16] One could think of the pre-rogative to not be resuscitated as an extension of the growing doctrine of informed consent. But in this case, the patient makes an informed refusal. She/he decides against resuscitation or other life-sustaining measures and removes consent for continued treatment.

Both the President's Commission report and expert guidelines on the care of the dying advanced by the Hastings Center in 1987[17] focused on the ethics of withholding and withdrawing life-sustaining therapy and *the negative right to be left alone*, if that were one's choice. These reports—and the scholarly literature during this period—maintained that decisions to withhold or withdraw life support were ethically equivalent. When these were the decisions of a patient or surrogate, then each decision was allowing nature to take its course. During this period bioethicists and philosophers distinguished the concepts of "killing and letting die."[18] Although practitioners might feel they had caused a patient to die when they removed a ventilator, bioethicists asserted and the law maintained that the discontinuation of life support was removing an impediment to death. The cause of death was not the removal of a ventilator but the underlying disease process that made the ventilator necessary in the first place.[19]

Quinlan and the Institutionalization of Hospital Ethics Committees

The Quinlan case was also important because it changed the hospital landscape by suggesting that ethical dilemmas in patient care were better addressed closer to the bedside and not in the courts. In its opinion, the New Jersey Supreme

Court suggested that alternative mechanisms be established to address ethical dilemmas in clinical practice and suggested a role for hospital ethics committees.[20] Hospital ethics committees first began to appear in the 1960s. Their initial concerns were the allocation of scarce resources like novel kidney dialysis machines and the ethical challenges posed by human subjects research.[21,22] These "forums for debate and resources for clinicians with difficult cases"[23]—to quote a description of the pioneering John Caldwell Fletcher—soon gained currency in clinical practice.

They were catalyzed by the Blue Ribbon Report of the President's Commission for the Study of Ethical Problems in Medicine and Biomedical and Behavioral Research that recommended that healthcare organizations have the responsibility:

> to ensure that there are appropriate procedures to enhance patients' competence, to provide for the designation of surrogates, to guarantee that patients are adequately informed, to overcome the influence of dominant institutional biases, to provide review of decision making, and to refer cases to the courts appropriately.[24]

The Commission urged the use of hospital-based ethics committees in order to spare the courts and keep decisions closer to the clinical context of care. Instead of an adversarial judicial forum for the resolution of conflict, the Commission suggested that "medical staff, along with the trustees and administrators of healthcare institutions, should explore and evaluate various formal and informal administrative arrangements for review and consultations, such as 'ethics committees.'"[25] By 1991 these recommendations had coalesced in requirements for hospital accreditation by the Joint Commission on Accreditation of Healthcare Organizations (JCAHO), which required the establishment of a mechanism for "the consideration of ethical issues arising in the care of patients and to provide education to caregivers and patients on ethical issues in health care."[23,26] This is now generally achieved through the use of ethics committees.

Cruzan and the Patient Self-Determination Act

The next major milestone in the evolution of bioethics and the right to die movement was the case of Nancy Beth Cruzan.[27] Like the Quinlan case, *Cruzan* involved a young woman in a vegetative state. But unlike *Quinlan, Cruzan* hinged on the removal of artificial nutrition and hydration. The lower courts in Missouri refused the family's request asserting that it would be improper to remove feedings unless there was unambiguous evidence of Ms. Cruzan's wishes.

Cruzan went all the way up to the US Supreme Court and became a landmark case. In its opinion, the Court recognized the constitutional *right* of a competent person to refuse life-sustaining therapy. The Court did not distinguish life-sustaining therapies, such as ventilators, from interventions, such as artificial nutrition and hydration. In all of these cases, patients could assert their self-determination and determine to which care they would consent.

Although this was an important judgment, the case was not a clear-cut victory for the proponents of patient self-determination. The *Cruzan* Court also asserted that each state could establish *evidentiary standards* or guidelines for decisions that involved surrogate decision makers. That is, when patients could not speak for themselves, the state could determine what amount of evidence of the patient's prior wishes would be necessary to grant authority to a surrogate to ask that care be withdrawn.[28] States could require *clear and convincing evidence*. Under this standard, the state would require specific evidence of what the patient said about life support. A lower evidentiary standard is called *substituted judgment*. When substituted judgment is invoked, decisions are informed by what is believed the patient would do under the prevailing circumstances. Here the surrogate places him/herself in the shoes of the patient and tries to make a decision as the patient might have, informed by knowledge of the patient's values and life experience. A final category is the *best interests* standard. This is a generic standard when nothing about the preferences of a particular patient are known. Here the issue is what sort of decision a reasonable person would make balancing benefits and burdens.

Missouri, in *Cruzan,* required clear and convincing evidence of the patient's prior wishes. Her parents asserted that they knew what their daughter would have wanted, but the Missouri courts maintained that they needed clear and convincing evidence of Ms. Cruzan's prior wishes in order to authorize an action that would lead to her death.[29] This presented a challenge to the family because like most young people Ms. Cruzan had not spoken about her wishes about the end of her life. At best, it seemed, the Cruzans were invoking a substituted judgment claim and asserting their right as parents to make a decision on behalf of the child that they had brought into the world.

So while the Supreme Court ruled that patients who were competent were permitted to refuse life-sustaining measures, the matter remained unsettled for the Cruzan family. The question still remained: was there enough evidence of Ms. Cruzan's wishes to allow the removal of the feeding tube? This issue was sent back down to the state courts in Missouri. Additional evidence of Ms. Cruzan's wishes was presented to a Missouri court and the removal of her feeding tube was authorized. She died on the day after Christmas 1990.

The difficulty of making end-of-life decisions without knowing what the patient would have wanted prompted Justice Sandra Day O'Connor to suggest a greater role for advance directives so that patients could articulate their preferences in advance of decision incapacity.[30] By completing an advance directive, which either laid out their preferences or designated someone to speak on their behalf, patients could ensure that their wishes would be followed if they could not speak for themselves.[31]

Influenced by Justice O'Connor's opinion, Senators Danforth of Missouri and Moynihan of New York introduced legislation to promote the use of advance directives.[32] Appropriate to an era marked by the rise of patient autonomy, this law was entitled the *Patient Self-Determination Act* (PSDA). It became law on December 1, 1991 and codified the rise of patient autonomy and the displacement of paternalism that had been evolving since Cardozo's ruling in the Schloendorff decision introduced the doctrine of informed consent.[33]

Advance Care Planning in Theory and Practice

Motivated by *Cruzan* and the new Patient Self-Determination Act, investigators in bioethics and health services research sought to study and better refine advance care planning. The largest and most important of these studies, the Study to Understand Prognoses and Preferences for Outcomes and Risks of Treatment (SUPPORT), suggested that there was a problem with advance care planning and, more generally, with how we die in America.[34]

Funded with $28 million from the Robert Wood Johnson Foundation, the SUPPORT study found that a disproportionate number of critically ill hospitalized patients received inadequate pain relief and that their preferences regarding end-of-life care were either unknown or ignored. Advance directives, at least as they were studied in their report,[35,36] were found to be ineffective in guiding care.

SUPPORT gained national attention and front page coverage in leading papers at a time when the nation was obsessed with questions of death and dying and best-selling books like Sherwin Nuland's *How We Die*[37] and the *Troubled Dream of Life* by Daniel Callahan, co-founder of the Hastings Center.[38] Ira Byock's elegiac *Dying Well,* which articulated a developmental approach to life completion and closure came a bit later, anticipating the broader emergence of hospice and palliative care.[39]

Against this cultural backdrop, the public read that advance directives did not work, that doctors ignored pain, and that physicians were often unaware of their patients' end-of-life care preferences.[40–41] SUPPORT's conclusions, both understood and misrepresented in the professional and lay press, led some to advocate for improved palliative care[42] and spurred others to work for the legalization of physician-assisted suicide. After all, if things were this bad in American hospitals, then patients must have an ability to control the timing and manner of their deaths.

From Self-Determination to Physician-Assisted Suicide

Writing about the passage of the Patient Self-Determination Act (PSDA), the physician ethicist Mark Siegler observed that moment in history represented the highwater mark of patient autonomy.[43] His prophetic comment anticipated the coming struggle that would follow in the wake of SUPPORT and the sad state of end-of-life care. How much control could be, or should be exerted to determine how we die? Were there limits to self-determination? How far did autonomy extend? When did the self-determination of the patient undermine the rights or well-being of others? These questions would dominate the nation's discourse only years after President George H. W. Bush signed the PSDA.

Simply put, the debate was whether the right to die and the right to refuse life-sustaining therapies extends, as well, to interventions that would hasten death. Proponents of physician-assisted suicide asserted that patients were entitled to a dignified end and the right to control the timing and manner of their death. They maintained that if patients had the right to refuse life-sustaining therapy, they also should be allowed to hasten their death through assisted suicide. The argument extending the patient's right to refuse life-sustaining therapy to a right to physician-assisted suicide struck many as taking patient self-determination too far.[44] Indeed some even asserted that it was a perversion of autonomy.[45]

In reality, physician-assisted suicide was more than a debate about a way to die. It encapsulated a growing cultural divide between those who wanted to exercise greater choice at the end of life and others who worried that the unrestrained rise of self-determination would erode traditional views about the sanctity of life. As we will see, this discussion played out on both coasts and in the heartland, in the federal courts in New York and Washington State, and in the media as the nation watched a crusading pathologist named Jack Kevorkian assist in the suicides of over one hundred individuals.[46] Ultimately, Oregon would legalize assisted suicide[47,48] and the US Supreme Court would maintain that there was not a constitutional right to such aid in dying though the court did not prohibit it in that state.

Physician-Assisted Suicide: Laying out the Arguments

To appreciate the complexity of the sociological forces that still influence care at the end of life, we need to review the major ethical arguments for and against assisted suicide in some detail. To do this we need to start with some definitions so we are clear about what we are actually discussing.

To begin with definitions, *euthanasia* comes from the Greek and literally means a good death.[49] Today the term is used to mean the intentional ending of a patient's life. In the past many clinicians would speak of passive and active euthanasia to describe what we now call the withholding or withdrawal of life-sustaining therapies.

In the old framework, *passive euthanasia* referred to decisions to let patients die without active intervention, such as resuscitation in the event of a cardiac arrest. Today we view this as allowing a patient to die or the withholding of life-sustaining therapy. Historically, *active euthanasia* referred to decisions to remove life-sustaining therapies such as a ventilator and allow nature to take its course. These cases are now termed withdrawals of care and not active euthanasia.

It is important to avoid the *passive* and *active euthanasia* terminology in clinical practice because it tends to conflate refusals of continued life-sustaining treatments with interventions, like assisted suicide, that can cause death to occur even when it is not inevitable.[50,51]

With this clarification in mind, we can now turn to the definition of physician-assisted suicide. Most commentators would define *physician-assisted suicide* (PAS) as when a physician knowingly provides a competent patient with the means to commit suicide. In physician-assisted suicide, the patient makes a voluntary request for this assistance. The patient then independently self-administers the lethal dose of medication. This contrasts with *voluntary active euthanasia* (VAE) when a physician provides *and* administers a lethal dose of medication to a patient who makes a voluntary request for such assistance.

Although PAS and VAE are in theory voluntary requests, the patient has less control when they do not themselves administer a lethal dose of medication. Voluntary active euthanasia is more open to becoming coerced or involuntary precisely because the physician controls medication administration. This lack of control raises the possibility that some acts of voluntary active euthanasia could be done without the patient's consent.

With these definitions in mind, one can think of a number of ethical positions that could be taken on the broader question of aid in dying.[52,53] The first is that PAS and VAE are morally wrong and thus proscribed. Individuals who advocate this point of view might argue that these actions are counter to a religious tradition or that they are inconsistent with their understanding of the ethos of the medical profession.[54–57] They are advocating a principled position against either PAS or VAE and would find no occasion in which either would be justifiable.

A second position maintains that although PAS and VAE might be acceptable in rare or exceptional circumstances, their legalization would be bad public policy and they should still not be permitted as public policy because they might lead to unintended and harmful consequences. Individuals who take this position may not find PAS or VAE inherently wrong but worry about them being abused in actual practice. An example of this position can be found in the actions of Governor Cuomo's Task Force on Life and the Law in New York. Although members of the Task Force were on record as favoring physician-assisted suicide, as a body they were unanimous in their opposition to a change in the law.[58]

The third position asserts that PAS is permissible and should be legalized. Proponents of this position draw the line on VAE because they fear that it can not be properly regulated.[59-61] This mixed position, in favor of PAS but opposed to VAE, has been proposed in multiple referendums across the United States and eventually was the basis for legalized physician-assisted suicide in Oregon.[62]

A final position would hold that both PAS and VAE are morally acceptable and that they should be legalized because they offer a benefit to individuals and society as a whole. Supporters of this position argue that competent individuals can invoke their self–determination to waive their right to life and that prohibiting this right would impose a constraint on one's rights and liberties.[63-66]

Physician-Assisted Suicide in the Courts

Arguments about patient rights and self-determination were to inform the courts' deliberations on physician-assisted suicide. Although the first case to come to public attention did not result in any enduring legal rulings, it did bring national attention to a more expansive right to die.

It could be said that the death of Janet Adkins catalyzed the debate that would eventually end up in the Supreme

Court. In June 1990, we read that Dr. Kevorkian had helped her die in the back of his now famous VW microbus. Adkins was a 54-year-old woman with a presumptive diagnosis of Alzheimer's disease.[67] She decided to be assisted in taking her own life after playing a game of tennis and writing a note to her family explaining her actions. She died connected to Dr. Kevorkian's suicide machine after depressing a switch that activated an injection of lethal medication.

An assisted suicide came from a more mainstream source when Timothy Quill of the University of Rochester School of Medicine wrote an essay that appeared in the *New England Journal of Medicine* in 1991.[65] He described how he assisted in the death of his long-time patient "Diane." Diane, a survivor of cervical cancer, had developed leukemia and chose to control the timing and manner of her death, even though there was a small chance that her second malignancy would not prove fatal. Quill's reflections in the nation's leading medical journal—coupled with Kevorkian's libertarian practices—led prominent physicians and medical ethicists to propose guidelines to legally regulate this practice.[61,68,69] If the practice were going on, they contended, better that it be regulated and open than occurring in an idiosyncratic fashion behind closed doors.

This desire for a legal mechanism for the conduct of this new practice eventually reached the federal courts. The first major case in federal court articulating the right to assisted suicide was one that involved a challenge to a provision in the State of Washington's law prohibiting physician-assisted suicide. The argument in favor of assisted suicide was a familiar one and hinged on the question of individual liberties and the right of the patient to have dominion over him/herself. In a historic decision a US District Court judge agreed.

Writing from Seattle, Judge Barbara Rothstein opined that, "There is no more profoundly personal decision, nor one which is closer to the heart of personal liberty, than the choice which a terminally ill person makes to end his or her suffering and hasten an inevitable death." [70,71] Analogizing to reproductive freedoms, she ruled that if women had the right to make important intimate choices about questions such as abortion, then dying patients—invoking liberty interests grounded in the 14th Amendment of the US Constitution—had a right to determine how they died.

About the same time another federal district judge ruled in the opposite direction. Timothy Quill, who had been Diane's doctor and had himself been brought up on charges of professional misconduct challenged New York State law prohibiting physician-assisted suicide. Although he had personally escaped sanction, his experiences led him to argue that the law violated the rights of patients to create their own destiny. This challenge of existing law failed in contrast to the Rothstein decision in Washington State. Citing the safety of the public and the risks of abuse, a federal judge in New York maintained that New York's ban on physician-assisted suicide was not unconstitutional.[72]

By the end of 1994, two federal courts of equal standing decided the same question differently. This split meant that these questions would be appealed and that they would ultimately end up in our highest courts. And that is what occurred.

On the West Coast, an initial decision in the Ninth Circuit Court overturned Judge Rothstein's decision. This reinstated Washington State's ban on physician-assisted suicide.[73] But given the volatility of the issue, this decision was appealed to all the judges on the circuit who took the unusual step of coming together to hear the case *en banc*. In this setting the Ninth Circuit Court decided that there *was* a constitutional right to physician-assisted suicide by an 8 to 3 margin. Writing for the majority, Judge Stephen Reinhardt again invoked the 14th Amendment. He asserted that, "A competent, terminally ill adult, having lived nearly the full measure of his life, has a strong liberty interest in choosing a dignified and humane death rather than being reduced to a state of helplessness, diapered, sedated, incompetent."[74]

Meanwhile in New York, the Second Circuit Court of Appeals reversed the district court's ruling. It found New York's ban on physician-assisted suicide unconstitutional. In their ruling the judges opined that New York's ban on physician-assisted suicide violated the *equal protection clause* of the 14th Amendment. The judges argued that if terminally ill patients had the right to have life-sustaining therapies withdrawn in order to die, then patients who were not sustained by such measures were denied an equal opportunity under the law to end their lives given the prohibition of physician-assisted suicide.[75,76]

With these two circuit decisions in place—and the state of the law in flux—the stage was set for a Supreme Court battle on this significant legal and ethical question. The Supreme Court heard the two cases together in January 1997.[77] That summer the Court ruled that there was not a constitutional right to physician-assisted suicide although they inferred a constitutional right to palliative care.[78] In addition, the Court distinguished pain relief from physician-assisted suicide, even if the use of opioid analgesia hastened death. (See section on the ethics of opioids, page 156-159).

At the same time the Supreme Court did not prevent individual states from being the "laboratory of democracy" and change their laws to permit assisted suicide if that was the will of the people.[79,80]

Several states availed themselves of this opportunity. From Maine to California, states had referendums asserting the right to physician-assisted suicide. Most were defeated by narrow margins. Oregon was the exception and its referendum was passed in November 1997. Implementation was held up but the Oregon Death with Dignity Act did go into effect in 1998. Under its provisions a physician could write a prescription for a lethal dose of medication if a terminally ill patient initiated a voluntary and repeated request for "assistance in dying." [81-84]

A Consensus on Palliative Care

If there were a silver lining about the physician-assisted suicide debate,[85] it was that this tension helped to catalyze the palliative care movement. Amidst the polarization over assisted suicide, the philosophy behind palliative care emerged as a compromise position. Its middle ground ethos of neither prolonging the dying process nor hastening death had broad secular and religious appeal.[86-88]

As the decade progressed, all but the most strident advocates or opponents of assisted suicide agreed to disagree on that contentious issue and work together to improve palliative care. This effort was supported by a number of philanthropies and by organized medicine.

In 1994 George Soros' Open Society Institute initiated the Project on Death in America to improve the care of the dying. A key feature of that initiative was a Faculty Scholars Program designed to support "outstanding clinicians, educators, and researchers in disseminating existing models of good care, developing new models for improving the care of the dying, and creating new approaches to the education of health professionals."[89] The Faculty Scholars Program has helped to develop a cohort of leaders in palliative care in over half of the nation's medical schools. Their reach has had a dramatic impact on medical education, clinical research, and, most critically, patient and family care.

In addition to the Soros initiative, the Robert Wood Johnson Foundation—the funder of SUPPORT—established its *Last Acts Project*. This was a coalition of prominent professional and lay organizations seeking to promote systemic reform of the "behavior of physicians and other health care providers, payers of care, hospitals and nursing homes, and consumers themselves."

Organized medicine has also played a role in improving end-of-life care. A milestone effort was a report on the care of the dying written by the Institute of Medicine. This seminal report articulated the normative expectation that "people with advanced, potentially fatal illness and those close to them should be able to expect and receive reliable, skillful and supportive care." To achieve this elusive goal, the panel made wide-ranging recommendations to improve professional competence, medical education, research and pain and symptom management. They urged that new resources be directed to finance the provision of palliative care and urged reform of restrictive drug prescription laws for opioid analgesia. Perhaps, most critically, they encouraged a public dialogue about our societal obligations to the dying and their families.[90]

A major focus of the Institute of Medicine report was the state of medical education for palliative care. The assessment of the quality of medical education was blunt. The writers observed that the clinical curriculum related to death and dying *"is conspicuous mainly by its relative absence."* [90] To respond to this dire situation the panel recommended a comprehensive response to these deficiencies that would foster basic competency in both the technical and humanistic dimensions of end–of–life care in all practitioners as well as the development of palliative care role models who could lead by example and expand the knowledge base in palliative medicine.[91]

In making many of these recommendations, the Institute of Medicine was following the innovative and pioneering initiative of the American Board of Internal Medicine (ABIM) to delineate core end-of-life care competencies for its trainees in post-graduate medical education.[92] It is encouraging to observe that since the ABIM's efforts in 1996, other professional organizations are making a systematic attempt to improve undergraduate, post-graduate, and continuing medical education in palliative care.[93-98]

Most notable among these efforts is Education for Physicians on End-of-Life Care (EPEC)—a continuing medical education program of the American Medical Association.[99] This initiative seeks to broaden the base of professional competence in end-of-life care by training local physician-leaders with a nationally developed curriculum so they can return to their communities and spearhead educational efforts. A parallel program, End-of-Life Nursing Education Consortium (ELNEC), has been developed for nursing education in palliative care.[100]

These initiatives were not limited to the national level but were complemented by significant activities in the states as well. By early 1998 at least 20 states had established commissions or task forces to study end-of-life care with at least six states (California, Colorado, Illinois, New Jersey, Tennessee, and Virginia) having their task forces established by law or a legislative resolution.[101]

The commission in New York deserves special mention because its origins and outcomes captured how much had been achieved and how much remains to be accomplished in end-of-life care. The commission was convened by then Attorney General Dennis Vacco after he had successfully argued against a constitutional right to assisted suicide, in *Quill v. Vacco*, before the US Supreme Court.[102] He had been urged to move beyond the rhetoric of opposition to constructively improve end-of-life care in his state.[103] His transformation from opponent of assisted suicide to advocate for palliative care was emblematic of the consensus that was evolving over the normative nature of palliative care. Unfortunately, the report was issued during the summer of 1998 when both Vacco and the Governor of New York were running for reelection. The report's release and recommendations were buried, as it were, for fear that the electorate would not really want to be upset by the difficult topic of death and dying. Vacco lost his bid for reelection.[104]

Back to the Future: The Schiavo Case

With all this progress in end-of-life care, it might come as a surprise that the nation was again gripped by a right to die case in the Fall of 2003. But that is precisely what happened in Florida when a federal court ruled that a feeding tube could be removed from Terri Schiavo, a 39-year-old woman in a chronic vegetative state following anoxic brain injury.[105] The case revealed lingering tensions between self-determination and the sanctity of life that had never fully been resolved in American life.

In a back to the future script, Schiavo was reminiscent of both *Quinlan* and *Cruzan*. Like *Quinlan, Schiavo* involved controversy over the diagnosis of the vegetative state. Like

Cruzan, it centered on the removal of a feeding tube from a patient who was vegetative and thus unable to provide her own consent.

Unlike *Quinlan* and *Cruzan, Schiavo* pitted a family against itself over questions of care. Mr. Schiavo, the patient's husband, had sought to remove his wife's feeding tube over the objections of her parents. He cited her prior wishes and the irreversibility of the vegetative state. The case had a long and complicated history in the courts. Multiple judges ruled that Mr. Schiavo was entitled to direct the patient's care. The courts heard the evidence and consistently recognized his authority to make decisions on behalf of his decisional incapacitated wife. The courts also determined that she was in a vegetative state based on expert unbiased testimony.

The Schindlers, Ms. Schiavo's parents, objected asserting that their daughter's wishes were not documented, documentation that would have been uncommon in 1990 when she became unconscious,[106] and that she had been misdiagnosed and still might recover. They released videotape to the media that showed her eyes open and blinking, with a fixed paretic smile. That these findings were entirely consistent with the wakeful unconsciousness of the vegetative state was open to rhetorical debate. Even though the vegetative state had been described three decades earlier and brought to the national stage in *Quinlan,* it again was open to discussion.[107] Amidst ideological opposition to the right to die, even Ms. Schiavo's diagnosis became a question of politics and not science. That this was described thirty-one years earlier and debated in *Quinlan* did not seem to matter. To many advocates of the right to life position, her diagnosis had taken on broader meaning as a value judgment. To them, clinical assessment had ceased to be a value-neutral exercise.[108]

This stance undermined the credibility of clinical assessment and allowed the public to weigh in and decide for themselves whether Ms. Schiavo was conscious or not. Untrained, many in the public were struck by the irony that one could be unconscious and still seem to be awake. And with this doubt they were susceptible to the Schindler's assertion that "starvation" might cause their daughter to suffer, even though suffering is not possible in a state of permanent unconsciousness.

Previously, the case was turned down by the US Supreme Court. The questions raised in *Schiavo* were settled by law. The *Cruzan* decision had established that adult competent patients could refuse life–sustaining therapy and surrogates could make decisions on their behalf according to provisions set out in state law. *Cruzan* had also determined that the refusal of artificial nutrition and hydration was no different than that of other life-sustaining therapies. As such, it too was constitutionally protected.

Despite these important precedents from the country's highest court, less than a week after Ms. Schiavo's feeding tube was removed, the Florida Legislature passed—and Governor Jeb Bush signed—a special bill authorizing him to make decisions on behalf of Ms. Schiavo.[109,110] This legislation was at the request of her parents.[111] So empowered, he ordered that the feeding tube be replaced. President Bush also publicly endorsed his brother's actions. Governor Bush's authority was the subject of legal challenge in the Florida Supreme Court which ruled that his actions were unconstitutional and a violation of the separation of powers.[112] The case was appealed to the US Supreme Court[113,114] but the Court refused to entertain the appeal, thus affirming the ruling of the Florida Supreme Court.[115]

Although the case of Terri Schiavo gained national attention in the Fall of 2003, the events of March 2005 gained a remarkable amount of national and international attention.[116] After the Florida Supreme Court ruled that Terri's Law was unconstitutional, the local trial court judge, George W. Greer, ordered that the tube be removed on March 18th. This set up a flurry of judicial appeals by the Schindler family and their allies in the right-to-life constituency. What resulted was the unprecedented involvement of the United States Congress in the drafting of a special act that would mandate review of the Schiavo case in federal court in order to ascertain whether there had been any violation of due process and Ms. Schiavo's civil rights.[117,118]

The proceedings in the House were carried on C-Span with physician-legislators playing an important role in offering their diagnostic impressions of Ms. Schiavo. They based their long-distance assessments on brief video snippets that were made available by the Schindlers. Central to the debate was whether Ms. Schiavo was accurately diagnosed as being in the permanent vegetative state and whether a person in that state could perceive the distress of "starvation."[119,120] Although her diagnosis had been adjudicated by the Courts, physician-members—including Senate Majority Leader Dr. Bill Frist—offered diagnostic assessments that were infused by ideology and departed from accepted clinical norms.[121-124] Important diagnostic distinctions amongst disorders of consciousness were confused and conflated.[125]

Congress passed the Act and President Bush returned from his Easter holiday in Crawford, Texas to sign the bill into law.[126] This intervention was hailed by pro-life advocates and decried by those who feared the intrusion of the state into the most private of matters and the erosion of federalism and the rule of law.[127-131] For review, the case went before US District Court Judge James D. Whittemore. He ruled as previous courts had and denied a request by the Schindler family to have the tube re-inserted.[132] His views were consistently upheld on appeal to the US Circuit Court and the US Supreme Court, both of which refused to hear the case.[133] Ms. Schiavo died on March 31st with her husband at her side 13 days after the feeding tube was removed.[134]

Epilogue

A final chapter in the Schiavo saga has been written. But even with this conclusion, it is almost certain that the after-life of Terri Schiavo will be a lingering cultural divide that will continue to influence decisions near the end of life. Although palliative care has gained a footing on our cultural landscape, we remain deeply split over questions of life and death. The divisions of the Schiavo-Schindler family reflect deeper national and what is often colloquially referred to as the Red State-Blue State divide.[135,136] Secular and religious influences continue to inform our perspective and our actions. Seemingly settled questions still linger beneath the surface and it would be naive to think that it were otherwise. We are intrigued by death, obsessed by its eventuality, ambivalent, anxious, and fearful. We want to master death through medical technology, control its timing and manner, deny our mortality, and affirm the value of the life we have been given.

If this history of the right to die serves any purpose, it should remind us that the care of the dying patient and his/her family is as much an exercise in sociology as medicine. Each clinical encounter occurs, whether we acknowledge it or not, against a cultural backdrop that needs to be appreciated to meet the needs of those entrusted to our care. When we think about end-of-life care, we should remind ourselves that each death continues to write the history of how we die in America. The story will long remain complex and nuanced. It is one worthy of continued study and clinical and intellectual engagement.

References

1 This discussion on the interplay of history, the law and decisions near the end-of-life is based upon and contains excerpts from: Fins JJ. Truth Telling and Reciprocity in the Doctor–Patient Relationship: A North American Perspective. In *Topics in Palliative Care* Volume 5. Bruera E and Portenoy RK, Eds. New York: Oxford University Press, 2001: pp. 81–94.

2 Montange CH. Informed Consent and the Dying Patient. *The Yale Law Journal* 83(8)(1974):1632–1664.

3 Zaubler TS, Viederman M, Fins JJ. Ethical, Legal, and Psychiatric Issues in Capacity, Competence, and Informed Consent: An Annotated Bibliography. *General Hospital Psychiatry* 18(1996):155–172.

4 *Salgo v. Leland Stanford Jr. Univ. Bd. of Trustees*, 317 P.2d 170 (Cal. Ct. App. 1957).

5 *Natanson v Kline*, 350 P 2d 1093, 1960.

6 *Canterbury v Spence*, 464 F 2d 772, 1972.

7 Annas G. Informed Consent, Cancer, and Truth in Prognosis. *New England Journal of Medicine* 330(1994):223–225.

8 Fins JJ. Constructing an Ethical Stereotaxy for Severe Brain Injury: Balancing Risks, Benefits and Access. *Nature Reviews Neuroscience* 4(2003):323–327.

9 Cranford RE. Medical Futility: Transforming a Clinical Concept into Legal and Social Policies. *Journal of the American Geriatrics Society* 42(1994):894–898.

10 Cantor NL. Twenty-five Years after Quinlan: A Review of the Jurisprudence of Death and Dying. *Journal of Law, Medicine & Ethics* 29(2)(2001 Summer):182–96.

11 *In re Quinlan*, 355 A 2d 647 (NJ 1976); *cert denied* 429 US 1992, 1976.

12 Jennett B and Plum F. Persistent Vegetative State after Brain Damage. A Syndrome in Search of a Name. *Lancet* 1(7753)(1972): 734–737.

13 Plum F and Posner J. *The Diagnosis of Stupor and Coma.* Philadelphia: F.A. Davis Company, 1983.

14 Plum, Fred. Personal Communication.

15 Annas GJ. The 'Right to Die' in America: Sloganeering from Quinlan and Cruzan to Quill and Kevorkian. *Duquesne Law Review* 34(4)(1996):875–897.

16 President's Commission for the Study of Ethical Problems in Medicine and Biomedical and Behavioral Research. *Deciding to Forego Life-Sustaining Treatment.* Washington, DC: US Government Printing Office, 1983.

17 The Hastings Center. *Guidelines on the Termination of Life Sustaining Treatment and the Care of the Dying.* Bloomington: Indiana University Press, 1987.

18 Brock D. Voluntary Active Euthanasia. *Hastings Center Report* 22(2)(1992):10–12.

19 Callahan D. Physician-Assisted Suicide: Opening the Door to Moral Mischief. *Newsday*, April 11, 1996.

20 This section draws from: Agrawal SK and Fins JJ. Ethics Committees and Case Consultation in the Hospital Setting. In *A Guide to Hospitals and Inpatient Care.* Siegler E, Mirafzali S, and Foust JB, Eds. New York: Springer, 2003.

21 Rothman DJ. *Strangers at the Bedside: a History of How Law and Bioethics Transformed Medical Decision Making.* New York: Basic Books, 1991.

22 Fletcher JC. Clinical Bioethics at NIH: History and a New Vision. *Kennedy Institute of Ethics Journal* 5(4)(1995):355–364.

23 Fletcher JC and Spencer EM. Ethics Services in Healthcare Organizations. In JC Fletcher, PA Lombardo, MF Marshall, FG Miller (Eds.). *Introduction to Clinical Ethics.* Frederick, MD: University Publishing Group, 1997.

24 Tulsky JA and Fox E. Evaluating Ethics Consultation: Framing the Questions. *Journal of Clinical Ethics* 7(2)(1996):109–115.

25 President's Commission for the Study of Ethical Problems in Medicine and Biomedical and Behavioral Research. *Deciding to Forego Life-Sustaining Treatment.* Washington, DC: US Government Printing Office, 1983.

26 Sexson WR and Thigpen J. Organization and Function of a Hospital Ethics Committee. *Clinics in Perinatology* 23(3)(1996):429–437.

27 *Cruzan v Director*, Missouri Department of Health, 110 S. Ct. 2841 (1990).

28 Sachs GA and Siegler M. Guidelines for Decision Making when the Patient is Incompetent. *Journal of Critical Illness* 6(1991):348–359.

29 Colby WH. *Long Goodbye, The Deaths of Nancy Cruzan*. Carlsbad, CA: Hay House, 2002.

30 Annas G. Nancy Cruzan in China. *Hastings Center Report* 20(5)(1990): 39–41.

31 Fins JJ. The Patient Self-Determination Act and Patient-Physician Collaboration in New York State. *New York State Journal of Medicine* 92(11)(1992):489–493.

32 McCloskey EL. The Patient Self-Determination Act. *Kennedy Institute of Ethics Journal* 1(2)(1991):163–169.

33 Zaubler TS, Viederman M, and Fins JJ. Ethical, Legal, and Psychiatric Issues in Capacity, Competence, and Informed Consent: An Annotated Bibliography of Representative Articles. *General Hospital Psychiatry* 18(3)(1996):155–172.

34 The SUPPORT Principal Investigators. A Controlled Trial to Improve Care for Seriously Ill Hospitalized Patients. *Journal of the American Medical Association* 274(20)(1995): 1591–1598.

35 Fins JJ. Advance Directives and SUPPORT. *Journal of the American Geriatrics Society* 45(1997):519–520.

36 Fins JJ. From Contract to Covenant in Advance Care Planning. *Journal of Law, Medicine & Ethics* 27(1)(1999):46–51.

37 Nuland S. *How We Die*. New York: Knopf, 1994.

38 Callahan D. *The Troubled Dream of Life: Living with Mortality*. New York: Simon and Schuster, 1993.

39 Byock I. *Dying Well: The Prospect for Growth at the End of Life*. New York: Riverhead Books, 1997.

40 Gilbert S. Doctors Often Fail to Heed the Wishes of the Dying Patient, *New York Times*, November 22, 1995, A1.

41 Colburn D. U.S. Patients' Dying Wishes Often Ignored, Study Finds Hospital Care Depersonalized, Resistant to Change, *Washington Post*, November 22, 1995, A1.

42 Sachs GA, Ahronhein JC, Rhymes JA, et al. Good Care of Dying Patients; The Alternative to Physician-assisted Suicide and Euthanasia. *Journal of the Amican Geriatrics Society* 43(5)(1995): 553–562.

43 Siegler M. Falling off the Pedestal: What Is Happening to the Traditional Doctor–Patient Relationship? *Mayo Clinic Proceedings* 68(5)(1993):401–467.

44 Callahan D. When Self-determination Runs Amok. *Hastings Center Report* 22(2)(1992):52–55.

45 Gaylin W and Jennings B. *The Perversion of Autonomy.* New York: The Free Press, 1996.

46 Belkin L. Doctor Tells of First Death Using his Suicide Device, *The New York Times,* June 6, 1990, A1.

47 *Oregon Death with Dignity Act,* Oregon Revised Statute, 127.800-127.897.

48 The Task Force to Improve the Care of Terminally-Ill Oregonians. *The Oregon Death with Dignity Act: A Guidebook for Health Care Providers.* Portland, OR: The Center for Ethics in Health Care, 1998.

49 *Shorter Oxford English Dictionary,* 5th ed., S.V. "euthanasia." Trumble WR, Brown L, Stevenson A, and Siefring J (Eds.). New York: Oxford University Press, 2002.

50 Miller FG, Fins JJ, and Snyder L. Assisted Suicide and Refusal of Treatment: Valid Distinction? *Annals of Internal Medicine* 132(6)(2000): 470–475.

51 Kamissar Y. In Defense of the Distinction Between Terminating Life Support and Actively Intervening to Promote or Bring About Death. *Journal of Biolaw & Business* 2(7&8)(1996):S:145–S:149.

52 Fins JJ and Bacchetta MD. Framing the Physician-Assisted Suicide and Voluntary Active Euthanasia Debate: The Role of Deontology, Consequentialism, and Clinical Pragmatism. *Journal of the American Geriatrics Society.* 43(5)(1995):563–568.

53 Fins JJ and Bacchetta MD. Physician Assisted Suicide and Euthanasia Debate: An Annotated Bibliography of Representative Articles. *Journal of Clinical Ethics* 5(4)(1994):329–340.

54 Pellegrino ED. Doctors Must Not Kill. *The Journal of Clinical Ethics* 3(2)(1992):95–102.

55 Kass LR. Death with Dignity & the Sanctity of Life. *Commentary.* March 1990: 33–43.

56 The Ramsey Colloquium. Always to Care, Never to Kill, *Wall Street Journal,* November 27, 1991.

57 Koop CE. The Challenge of Definition. *Hastings Center Report* 19(1)(1989):2–3.

58 New York State Task Force on Life and the Law. *When Death is Sought: Assisted Suicide and the Constitution.* State of New York, 1994.

59 Clouser KD. The Challenge for Future Debate on Euthanasia. *Journal of Pain and Symptom Management* 6(5)(1991):306–311.

60 Battin MP. Euthanasia: The Way We Do It. The Way They Do It. *Journal of Pain and Symptom Management* 6(5)(1991):298–305.

61 Quill TE, Cassel CK, and Meier DE. Care of the Hopelessly Ill—Proposed Criteria for Physician Assisted Suicide. *New England Journal of Medicine* 327(19)(1992): 1380–1384.

62 Fins JJ. Physician Assisted Suicide and the Right to Care. *Cancer Control: Journal of the Moffitt Cancer Center* 3(3)(1996):272–278.

63 Humphry D and Wickett A. *The Right to Die.* Eugene, OR: The Hemlock Society, 1990.

64 Humphry D. *Final Exit: The Practicalities of Self-Deliverance and Assisted Suicide for the Dying.* Eugene, OR: Hemlock Society, 1991.

65 Quill TE. Death and Dignity: A Case of Individualized Decision Making. *New England Journal of Medicine* 324(10)(1991):691–694.

66 Quill TE. *Death and Dignity: Making Choices and Taking Charge.* New York: W.W. Norton, 1993.

67 Belkin L. Doctor Tells of First Death Using his Suicide Device, *New York Times,* June 6, 1990, A1.

68 Miller FG and Fletcher JC. The Case for Legalized Euthanasia. *Perspectives in Biology and Medicine* 36(2)(1993):159–176.

69 Miller FG, Quill TE, Brody H, et al. Regulating Physician-Assisted Death. *New England Journal of Medicine* 331(2)(1994):119–123.

70 *Compassion in Dying v. Washington,* 850 F. Supp. 1455 (W.D. Wash. 1994).

71 Egan T. Federal Judge Says Ban on Suicide Aid is Unconstitutional, *New York Times,* May 5, 1994, A1.

72 *Quill v. Koppel,* 94 Civ. 5321.

73 *Compassion in Dying v. Washington,* No. 94-35534 (9th Cir.) March 9, 1995; 1995 US App. LEXIS 4589.

74 1996 WL 94848 9th Cir. (Wash).

75 1996 U.S. App. Lexis 62115,*37.

76 Fins JJ. What Medicine and the Law should do for the Physician-Assisted Suicide Debate. *CCAR Journal* 44(2)(1997):46–53.

77 Transcript of Oral Arguments before the US Supreme Court. Justices Hear Arguments on Laws Barring Physician-assisted Suicide. *Chicago Daily Law Bulletin* Vol. 143, No. 7, January 10, 1997.

78 Burt RA. The Supreme Court Speaks—Not Assisted Suicide but a Constitutional Right to Palliative Care. *New England Journal of Medicine* 337(17)(1997):1234–6.

79 Transcript of Oral Arguments before the US Supreme Court. Justices Hear Arguments on Laws Barring Physician-assisted Suicide. *Chicago Daily Law Bulletin* Vol. 143, No. 7, January 10, 1997.

80 *Vacco v Quill* No. 95-1858, 1997 U.S. Lexis 40388 and *State of Washington v. Glucksberg* No. 96-110, 1997 U.S. Lexis 4039.

81 *Oregon Death with Dignity Act*, Oregon Revised Statute 127.800-127.897.

82 Fins JJ. Physician-Assisted Suicide and the Right to Care. *Cancer Control* 3(3)(1996):272-278.

83 The Task Force to Improve the Care of Terminally-Ill Oregonians. *The Oregon Death with Dignity Act: A Guidebook for Health Care Providers.* Portland, OR: The Center for Ethics in Health Care, 1998.

84 Chin AE, Hedberg K, Higginson GK, Fleming DW. Legalized physician-assisted Suicide in Oregon—The First Year's Experience. *New England Journal of Medicine* 340(7)(1999):577-83.

85 Lee MA and Tolle SW. Oregon's Assisted Suicide Vote: The Silver Lining. *Annals of Internal Medicine* 124(2)(1996):267-269.

86 Foley KM. Competent Care for the Dying Instead of Physician-assisted Suicide. *New England Journal of Medicine* 336(1)(1997):54-58.

87 Sachs GA, Ahronhein JC, Rhymes JA, et al. Good Care of Dying Patients: The Alternative to Physician-Assisted Suicide and Euthanasia. *Journal of the American Geriatrics Society* 43(5)(1995): 553-562.

88 McCabe MJ. *The Hospice Movement—An Alternative to Euthanasia. Pars Dissertatio ad Doctoratum in Theolgia Morali Consequendum.* Dal Vicariato di Roma, 1994.

89 Project on Death in America. *Report of Activities: July 1994–December 1997.* New York: Open Society Institute, 1998.

90 Field MJ and Cassel CK, Eds. *Approaching Death: Improving Care at the End of Life.* Washington, DC: Committee on Care at the End of Life, Institute of Medicine-National Academy Press. 1997.

91 Field and Cassel, 207-234.

92 American Board of Internal Medicine. *Caring for the Dying: Identification and Promotion of Physician Competency.* Philadelphia: ABIM, 1996.

93 Billings JA and Block S. Palliative Care in Undergraduate Medical Education: Status Report and Future Directions. *Journal of the American Medical Association.* 278(9)(1997):733-8.

94 The Medical School Objectives Writing Group. Learning Objectives for Medical Student Education—Guidelines for Medical Schools: Report I of the Medical School Objectives Project. *Academic Medicine* 74(1)(1999):13-18.

95 Meekin SA, Klein JE, Fleischman AR, and Fins JJ. Development of a Palliative Education Assessment Tool for Medical Student Education. *Academic Medicine* 75(10)(2000):986-992.

96 Wood EB, Meekin SA, Fins JJ and Fleischman, AR. Enhancing Palliative Care Education in Medical School Curricula: Implementation of the Palliative Education Assessment Tool. *Academic Medicine* 77(4)(2002):285-291.

97 Block, SD, Bernier GM, Crawley LM, et al. *Incorporating Palliative Care into Primary Care Education.* Developed for the National Consensus Conference on Medical Education for Care Near the End of Life. *Journal of General Internal Medicine.* 13(11)(1998):768–73.

98 Weissman DE and Griffie J. Integration of palliative medicine at the Medical College of Wisconsin 1990–1996. *Journal of Pain and Symptom Management.* 15(3)(1998):195–201.

99 American Medical Association. *EPEC-Education for Physicians on End-of-Life Care.* Chicago: American Medical Association, 1998.

100 Sherman DW, Matzo ML, Rogers S, et al. Achieving Quality Care at the End of Life: A Focus on the End-of-Life Nursing Education Consortium (ELNEC) Curriculum. *Journal of Professional Nursing* 18(5)(2002): 255–262.

101 Merritt D, Fox-Grage W, Rothouse M, Lynn J, Cohn F, Forlini JH. State Initiatives in End-of-Life Care: Policy Guide for State Legislators. Washington, DC: National Conference of State Legislatures and The Center to Improve Care of the Dying, 1998.

102 Attorney General Dennis C. Vacco's Commission on Quality Care at the End of Life. *Final Report.* New York: July 1998.

103 Foley, Kathleen M. Personal Communication.

104 Edited excerpts on the culture of death and dying in America have been taken from: Fins JJ. Death and Dying in the 1990s: Intimations of Reality and Immortality. *Generations: Journal of the American Society on Aging* 23(1)(1999):81–86.

105 Wallis C. The Twilight Zone of Consciousness. *Time*, October 27, 2003, 43–44.

106 Fins JJ. Letter to the Editor re: A Patient's Wishes and 'Terri's Law.' *New York Time*, September 7, 2004, A-22.

107 MacKeen D and Rabin R. States of Awareness. *Newsday*, October 26, 2003.

108 Fins JJ and Plum F. Neurological Diagnosis is More than a State of Mind: Diagnostic Clarity and Impaired Consciousness. *Archives of Neurology* 61(9)(2004):1354–1355.

109 US Senate Bill No. HB 35-E.

110 Charatan F. Governor Jeb Bush Intervenes in Right to Die Case. *British Medical Journal* 327 (7421)(2003):949..

111 Reuters. Parents Ask Florida Gov. to Save Comatose Daughter, *New York Times*, October 13, 2003.

112 Supreme Court of Florida. No. SC04-925 Jeb Bush, Governor of Florida, et al., Appellants, vs. MICHAEL SCHIAVO, Guardian of Theresa Schiavo, Appellee. September 23, 2004.

113 In the Circuit Court for Pinellas County, Florida. Circuit Civil Case No. 03-008212-CI-20. Michael Schiavo, Petitioner as Guardian of the person of Theresa Maria Schiavo vs. Jeb Bush, Governor of the State of Florida and Charlie Crist, Attorney General of the State of Florida, Respondents.

114 Goodnough A. Comatose Woman's Case Heard by Florida court, Law Passed to Prolong Life Is at Issue. *The New York Times*, 7 September 2004, A-14.

115 Long P. Supreme Court Refuses to Take Governor's Appeal in Schiavo Case. *Miami Herald* website *http://www.miami.com/mld/miamiherald/news/breaking_news/10721955.htm?1c*. Accessed January 24, 2005.

116 Annas GJ. "Culture of Life" Politics at the Bedside—The Case of Terri Schiavo. *New England Journal of Medicine*. March 23, 2005. [Epub ahead of print]

117 Hulse C and Kirkpatrick DD. Congress Passes and Bush Signs Schiavo Measure. *The New York Times*. March 21, 2005, A-1.

118 Kirkpatrick DD and Stolberg SG. How Family's Cause Reached the Halls of Congress. *The New York Times*. March 22, 2005, A-1.

119 Wilson JQ. Killing Terri. *The Wall Street Journal*. March 21, 2005, A-16.

120 Schwartz J. Neither 'Starvation' nor Suffering It Connotes Applies to Schiavo, Doctors Say. *The New York Times*. March 25, 2005, A-14.

121 Jennett B. *The Vegetative State*. Cambridge: Cambridge University Press, 2002.

122 Interview of Joseph J. Fins, M.D., by Elizabeth Kaledin. CBS Evening News. March 21, 2005.

123 Interview of Joseph J. Fins, M.D. by Dr. David Marks. WCBS-TV News. March 22, 2005.

124 Stolberg S. Drawing Some Criticism, Legislators with Medical Degrees Offer Opinions on Schiavo Case. *The New York Times*. March 23, 2005, A-14.

125 Fins JJ. Rethinking Disorders of Consciousness: New Research and Its Implications. *The Hastings Center Report* 35(2)(2005):22–24.

126 Bumiller E. Supporters Praise Bush's Swift Return to Washington. *The New York Times*. March 21, 2005, A-15.

127 Interview of Joseph J. Fins, M.D. CNN, Lou Dobbs Tonight. March 21, 2005.

128 Fried C. Federalism Has a Right to Life, Too. *The New York Times*. March 23, 2005, A-17.

129 Gilgoff D. Life and Death Politics. *U.S. News & World Report.* April 4, 2005, pp. 15–21.

130 Interview of Joseph J. Fins, M.D. PRI/NPR Radio, To the Point. March 21, 2005.

131 New York Times Editorial. Exploiting Terri Schiavo, A Blow to the Rule of Law. *The New York Times,* A-22.

132 Goodnough A. U.S. Judge Denies Feeding-Tube Bid in Schiavo's Case. *The New York Times.* March 23, 2005, A-1.

133 Goodnough A. Supreme Court Refuses to Hear the Schiavo Case. *The New York Times.* March 25, 2005, A-1.

134 Goodnough A. Schiavo Dies, Ending Bitter Case Over Feeding Tube. *The New York Times.* April 1, 2005, A-1.

c h a p t e r   f o u r

End-of-Life Care in the Hospital

Death in the Modern Hospital

The complex sociology of death and dying and caregiving has its nexus in the acute care hospital. For most of us, the hospital will be the intersection of societal forces and personal loss. Sixty percent of all deaths occur in the hospital and, for better or worse,[1] most of your training about end-of-life care will occur in that setting.[2] In this chapter we will consider how the organization of the hospital influences the care of the dying, review end-of-life practice patterns in that setting, and consider the challenge of palliative care in this context.

The origins of the modern hospital are relatively recent. They date to early twentieth century when advances in surgical technique required facilities not available in the private

homes of surgeons. The modern hospital developed to provide a setting for the use of more sophisticated technology
and has been described as the work place of the surgeon, a
phrase which epitomizes acute interventions and rescue by
dramatic and highly technological innovations.[3]

The development of the modern hospital transformed
where death would occur.[4] As the century progressed,
patients would no longer die in their homes surrounded by
family. Instead, death would increasingly occur in the acute
care setting of the hospital within an institutional culture that
emphasized the medical imperative of rescue and cure.

Medical Rescue and Intensive Care

This ethos of rescue and cure pervades the modern hospital
but is most evident in the intensive care unit, the setting for
over 40 percent of deaths of hospitalized patients.[5] Over half
of dying patients will pass through the ICU during their terminal admission and receive aggressive life-sustaining interventions like ventilatory support and medications for blood
pressure support. The ICU clearly influences the care of
patients who pass through its doors but it would be a mistake to think that only these patients are influenced by the
sort of care provided in the ICU. The culture of intensive
care, with its emphasis on technology and specialization,
stretches beyond its own walls with the ICU as a central and
organizing fixture of hospital practice.[6]

It must be said that many have benefited from the technology and expertise that resides in the intensive care unit
with its emphasis on saving or prolonging life. But it also
must be acknowledged that the good done there is tempered

when the ICU becomes a site for the care of patients who are in the process of dying. In the face of end-stage disease, these patients are often over-treated, subjected to poor pain management, and deprived of contact with family as death approaches. Surveys of ICU patients rated arterial blood gases as severely painful; mechanical ventilation, nasogastric tubes, central line placement and peripheral IV placement as moderately painful; and urethral catheters, intramuscular injections, and mechanical restraints as minimally painful.[7,8] These errors of omission and commission are not intentional but reflect deep cultural forces in modern medicine, which are especially prominent in intensive care.[9]

Because of the complexity of illness and the emphasis placed on saving or prolonging life, clinicians in the ICU tend to adopt a reductive focus on the patient's organ systems, on quantitative results of diagnostic tests, and on technological procedures to combat disease.[10] Care is so nuanced that it is divided into ever-smaller parts. The needs of the whole person, not to mention the family, are subsumed by attention to the settings on a ventilator, the latest blood gas, or the newest antibiotic added to a long list of medications.

Teams of physicians can be seen rounding with flow sheets, which organize the patient's physiology. They round in a space designed for the provision of technologically advanced care. The environment can often be sterile and stark in appearance. Patient rooms lack the privacy conducive to intimate family contact and there is often no designated, private space for communication between clinicians and family members who must speak for incapacitated patients.

Everything in the unit is mobile. The equipment, beds, supply carts, and equipment are all portable and on rollers, suggesting transience and a lack of permanence which convey a sense of perpetual motion.[11] And the staff is in perpetual motion rushing to pursue clinical details that are always challenging. In this setting it is often difficult for practitioners to step back from the prevailing rescue orientation to review the goals of treatment, incorporating realistic assessments of patient prognosis or the preferences of the patient and family. There often is not time.[12] Clinicians are on a frantic pace and care is often tactical responding to one crisis after another. There is little time for strategy and thinking about the bigger picture.

But time is not the only factor. Too often, the culture of intensive care promotes and rewards diagnostic acumen and technical competence at the expense of communication. The result is that patients and family may feel bewildered and isolated at a time of crisis.

Consider the example of a patient with widely metastatic breast cancer who is ventilator dependent because of pneumonia and who has developed acute renal failure of unknown etiology. A nephrologist is consulted and determines the diagnosis. It is a subtle diagnosis but still an irreversible cause of renal failure. The nephrologist takes that in stride and initiates dialysis for fluid overload and metabolic acidosis. He is now on autopilot. The line-placement is routine. His mind is elsewhere pleased with his diagnostic skills and flattered by an invitation to do "Professor's Rounds" later in the week. The tragedy of the patient's worsening condition is less important than the peer recognition garnered from making a complex diagnosis.

Following the procedure, the patient has more acceptable electrolytes. The nephrologist tells the family that the dialysis was "successful." "We got a couple of liters of fluid off and the bicarbonate is back to normal." The patient's husband thanks the nephrologist for his efforts and is buoyed by the promising news. No one has mentioned that the patient has irreversible kidney damage and that dialysis will be a permanent fixture in his wife's ever-shortening life. He will learn that in a couple of days when he is surprised to find dialysis technicians returning to cleanse his wife's blood once again. He did not appreciate that the kidney damage was permanent. "I thought the dialysis was successful," he says to one of the techs.

He was surprised because he rightly assumed that all the members of the team were communicating and on the same page, that all information would be shared so that everyone would be aware of the goals and plans and that they would effectively work together. Too often this is not the case. Pieces of information may be known to some, but not others. Physicians discuss the clinical condition and the course of treatment. The nurse sees firsthand the patient's response to treatment, but may not have heard the conversation on morning rounds about prognosis. The social worker is considering the family dynamics, religious/cultural issues, and financial matters in the context of discharge planning and psychosocial support. The clerk may be the only one who has actually seen the advance directive, since she placed it in the medical record.[13]

Even if all of this information were documented in the medical record, it may not be known to all. Different readers focus on different aspects of the information, and team members may not take the time to read each other's notes. The very nature and structure of the ICU and modern hospital care rely upon the expertise of many, but staffing and time constraints can make it seem difficult, sometimes impossible, to achieve any kind of interdisciplinary approach to care.

Returning to our case, it is important to note that the husband had received partial truths. The "good news" shared by the nephrologist was positive at some level. Death by renal failure had been dodged with dialysis. But death from another cause had not been averted, only delayed. The family who heard that dialysis was "successful" was especially vulnerable because of their heartfelt desire for good news. They were unable to see renal failure as additional evidence of the patient's terminal condition.

This prognostic information is not shared with the family by the nephrologist for a number of reasons. First, he is constrained by a sort of professional etiquette. He is a consultant and not the patient's primary attending physician. Under seemingly Victorian rules, he works at the behest of the attending physician who asked for the consultation. Any global statements about prognosis, future care, and overall strategy are the attending's to make. Second, he may not be all that familiar with the larger picture of the patient's care. He was contacted to assess the patient for acute renal failure and to initiate dialysis if needed. That done, he had done his job. Given his unfamiliarity with the case and his deference to the attending physician, who knows the patient best, he is relieved of the burden of engaging the big issues of death and dying. As a consultant, it would indeed be inappropriate to have a more global conversation.

This deference is not limited to nephrology but to the other specialists who participate in the case. Each will comment on their particular organ system, the numbers that reflect its status, and the intervention that is proposed to correct the situation. Often it does not matter that the overall prognosis of the patient is dire and that attempts to ameliorate physiologic derangements will only prolong an inevitable death. Each clinician seems to operate in their own silo, sequestered from each other save for their collective notes in the chart.

While there may be many reasons for this, one factor is likely to be the clinicians' death anxiety and own discomfort with open discussion.[14,15] They may avoid difficult conversations. The retreat to the specialized realm of physiology is also protective. This allows them to speak in technical language instead of addressing more emotionally charged issues like prognosis or life expectancy,[16] the real questions on everyone's mind. Another, more basic reason may simply be that they were never trained to have conversations about end-of-life care.

In this case, the primary care attending who knows the patient best is no longer the attending of record because the patient is in the ICU. That role is taken by the ICU attending who is more technically skilled about the life-sustaining therapies employed there. Although many intensivists bring great humanism and technical expertise to the care of critically ill patients,[17] each must contend with the complexity of the patient's illness while being hampered by the fact that they knew neither patient nor family prior to admission to the unit. So while they have the technological knowledge to manage the patient's disease, they may be less able to manage the broader consequences of her illness.

And so it goes. Communication can become so fragmented that no one is really in charge. This is captured in an often-quoted remark of Dr. Eugene Stead, the longtime chairman of medicine at Duke University School of Medicine. Commenting on the confusion that can occur when everyone is involved but no one seems to be in charge, Dr. Stead observed, "what this patient needs is a doctor." [18] By that, Dr. Stead was commenting on the fragmentation of the doctor–patient/family relationship that can often complicate the care of the severely ill patient.

This fragmentation can lead to disputes between members of the clinical team and with the patient and family in the ICU setting.[19] This can be bewildering to families who need more guidance, not less, given the complexity of the care provided in that setting. But ultimately, there is a greater premium on the provision of technically excellent care than excellent communication.[20]

Fostering Communication

If palliative care is about making choices, then these choices need to be adequately communicated to patients and families in a timely fashion. Without knowing that palliative care is an option it cannot be selected as a care strategy. Neither will it be chosen if it is devalued in interactions that betray a bias to cure over care, even when cure is elusive and unlikely.

As our case illustrates, communication is a most important catalyst for the selection of palliation. Indeed, poor communication renders all other medical care ineffective. Without effective communication, palliative care will remain an unstated option. At worst, it can be one that is discounted.[21] This might be through a careless phrase like, "Well, we could *just* palliate." Here the adverb, *just*, betrays a bias that palliative care is something less valuable than other care strategies. Subtly, a patient or family might make a judgment that palliative care is a substandard default option, not the sort of care to which they or a loved one is entitled. Or, they may feel abandoned if they choose palliative care. It does not matter that palliative care is effective in pain and symptom management and that curative interventions will be futile in terminal illness.[22] Considered this way, communication—not opioid analgesia—becomes the central catalyst to effective palliative care. And so we need to spend some time looking at why communication can be such a challenge in the hospital setting.

In the complex setting of a hospital, with so many involved in the provision of care, good communication is emblematic of understanding, caring, and trust. As such, it is also the foundation of the doctor–patient relationship. From diagnostic determinations to treatment options, it is critical to both doctor and patient that information is shared and understood on a continuing basis. Without good communication, doctors may miss important medical or personal elements of the patient's "story." Patients may not be able to understand clinical information upon which informed decisions about their own medical care is based.

Patients and families also expect physicians to listen to them as they express their concerns, fears, beliefs, and to initiate conversations about their illness, treatments, quality of life, and death and dying.[23] They expect the physician to incorporate knowledge and understanding of each individual into the treatment plan, and not just focus on the disease. The information being exchanged is a valuable commodity; the more you know, the more effective you can be as a clinician.

Beside the physical impact of disease and hospitalization, patients often feel robbed of any sense of control over their lives.[24] Since most of us define ourselves through our responsibilities and relationships, it is a devastating blow to find that life is now defined by hospital routines, tests, and treatments that dictate what happens and when. Ongoing communication with the clinician can help the patient feel more in control, appreciate options, and understand the reasons and timing for each intervention. Furthermore, when the patient has the opportunity to inform clinicians about her values, it fosters the feeling that her individuality is being recognized and acknowledged. The loss of these opportunities for discussion can result in a profound sense of isolation, anonymity, and abandonment.

Communication, Palliation, and the Road Not Taken

Communication in the hospital is especially important because that is where critical decisions are made. Decisions to pursue palliative care can be precipitated by hospitalization or a change in the course of illness during hospitalization. These events become critical transition points where options diverge and paths are chosen. They can be opportunities for conversations and informed decision making *if* choices are presented for consideration. But that does not always take place.

Perhaps a metaphor would be helpful here to convey what we mean. Imagine that the acute care setting of the hospital is like an interstate highway and that hospice and palliative care is the country road that rambles along side the interstate. Like a hospital, the interstate loves its technology. Cars, of ever increasing size and complexity, speed along. Like the ICU we just described, everything is highly mobile. There is no permanence; cars are swept along. Everyone has to drive at a minimum speed to keep up. Speeds are quick and accidents are frequent and sometimes life-threatening. Gas is guzzled and, as in the hospital, resources like blood products and antibiotics are consumed.

Like choices in the hospital, for those on the interstate there are a number of key decision points and often a sense of no turning back if the "wrong" choice is made. On the interstate, the choice is when to exit. But the exits—and rest stops—are widely spaced. If you miss your exit, you may have to travel fifty miles until the next one appears, in that you may be in urgent need of some coffee or a rest room. In this context, palliative care is the adjoining country road sometimes seen from the highway but still far away. It is a rambling road marked by weeping willows growing next to a little brook and a charming white house with green shutters, which might metaphorically represent hospice care. The house, like hospice, is out of the mainstream—on a path not taken—if you missed the opportunity to exit from the interstate.

People who travel on that country road are not concerned with reaching the elusive cure at road's end. Rather, they travel along, enjoying the scenery, stopping now and then to admire a view, to rest in the shade of a grove of trees. The patient on the highway periodically catches a glimpse of this alternative route and admires its peaceful atmosphere, but isn't sure it is time to exit. Just as he considers turning off the highway and abandoning the struggle for a cure to travel the more peaceful, leisurely path, the exit ramp whizzes by. The patient wasn't prepared for the exit and could not turn off. The patient realizes that he must continue along the highway for a while longer, falsely consoled by the faint prospect that the highway may lead to a cure. The highway of aggressive medical treatment runs fast, is heavily traveled, but can lack landmarks and the signage necessary to know when it is time to make for the exit ramp and the winding country road representing palliative care. These signs are there and it is your responsibility to communicate them to patients and families.

Milestones at the End of Life

If we hope to guide patients and families as they make their final journey, it is necessary to appreciate the sequence of end-of-life decision making and the usual patterns that occur during the patient's terminal phase of illness. My work in ethics case consultation[25,26,27,28] and empirical studies of end-of-life practice patterns, conducted with colleagues,[5,6] has led to a sense of the sequence of decisions made at the end of life. Although this construct was informed by the American context of care, investigators in Australia using our methodology have identified similar practice patterns there.[29] This knowledge has assisted us in guiding patients and families through this unfamiliar territory and helped to prevent disputes and contentious miscommunication.

There is a roadmap at the end of life with identifiable milestones that can help inform communication and care strategies. In a retrospective study of end-of-life practice patterns among adult patients, we found that there is a normative progression or sequence of decision making. We sought to understand when patients were made DNR, when clinicians felt that death was imminent, and when comfort care plans were initiated.

Our first observation, confirmed by many others, is that little advance care planning occurs even up to the admission when the patient will die. Only 28 percent of patients had a durable power of attorney or health care proxy prior to admission. Only 13 had a DNR order before entering the hospital. These numbers are rather low when one considers that our sample only included patients who would soon die. This indicates that there is an ongoing expectation for cure, even late into the course of illness.

Contrary to popular convention, we found that the completion of a DNR order was the *first* major end-of-life decision. This was later followed by evidence that the clinicians considered the patient to be dying and by the institution of comfort measures.

During this sequence, 77 percent of patients had a DNR order prior to death. This rose to 90 percent with those patients who had a length of stay over three weeks. Only 32 percent of patients consented to their own DNR orders. Most DNR orders, (64 percent), were agreed to by surrogates after the patient had lost decision-making capacity. So to return to our highway metaphor, the loss of decision-making capacity can be viewed as an important sign that the end is approaching.

Loss of capacity, often with a loss of consciousness, is a major prognostic indicator in dying patients. Once the patient has become unconscious, surrogates may feel more willing to forego resuscitation and pursue less aggressive care. Surrogates may be more hopeful if the patient remains awake and interactive even in the setting of impaired decision-making capacity.

In our study, the average length of stay was 16.9 days, with a median stay of 9.0 days. Given this median duration of admission, DNR orders were written—on median—two days after admission. Patients were then identified as dying at 4.5 days. A comfort care plan was noted 6.0 days after admission. If we consider this data as time *prior* to death, patients were identified as dying 3.5 days prior to death and received comfort care 2.0 days prior to death. This data might be said to capture the prevailing notion that the provision of palliative care was "too little and too late."[30] While 77 percent of patients were DNR, only 72 percent were identified as dying and just 46 percent received a comfort plan.

This sequence from DNR order to being identified by staff as dying to the provision of comfort care plans is an important one to understand. In our view it represents the evolution of a moral consensus that helps patients, families, and clinicians make the transition from aggressive curative care to palliative care. The initial DNR order is a weak moral consensus between clinician and surrogate that life-sustaining technology will not be used *if* the patient has a respiratory or cardiac arrest. That is, the decision to forego aggressive care is contingent upon an intervening catastrophic event. That event would legitimate a decision to withhold care even though a consensus has not yet emerged to withdraw life-sustaining interventions like a ventilator.

The next nodal point in this sequence is the determination by someone on the clinical team that the patient is dying. In our study, we carefully defined what sort of language would be necessary to indicate that a patient had been identified in the medical record as dying.

A notation in the chart that the patient is dying is no guarantee that they will receive comfort care. A consensus needs to develop amongst all the stakeholders that the patient is dying. This realization generally follows the initial DNR designation and represents a growing appreciation of a patient's dire prognosis. Once that is accepted by the team, and most critically by the attending physician in charge, the family can be approached about comfort care.

The complexity of this evolution and the need for broad consensus among both professional and lay decision makers helps explain why this process takes so long, a mean of 15 days after admission, as compared to an overall length of stay of 17 days. It also explains why just 46 percent of patients were designated to receive comfort measures during their terminal admission and the elasticity of "comfort care" at the end of life.

In our study, the provision of comfort care in the hospital appears to lack a consistent focus. Only 13 percent of those on a ventilator and 19 percent receiving artificial nutrition and hydration were withdrawn from these life-sustaining therapies prior to death. In addition, significant proportions of patients designated to receive "comfort care" continued to receive non-comfort measures: 13 percent remained on a ventilator, 11 percent received artificial nutrition and hydration, 30 percent had continued blood draws for diagnostic testing, and 41 percent received antibiotics. This variance in practice indicates the difficulty of doing less and letting go. It suggests that even late into the course of illness there is ambivalence about potential outcomes and adherence to hospital routines, like blood draws, even though the information obtained may not be directed to any therapeutic intervention.

Ambivalence and Medical Futility

The evolution to a comfort care plan will not occur if there is disagreement or if members of the team are not communicating well with each other. The communication challenge can be especially problematic if the observation that the patient is dying comes from a junior member, like a nurse or house officer.[31] Although these clinicians are moral agents, their opinions can be discounted by more senior staff.[32]

Agreement to comfort care measures, unlike the earlier DNR order, suggests a greater acceptance that death is imminent because a decision to pursue less aggressive care is not contingent upon an intervening catastrophic event like a cardiac arrest. The patient's course has already progressed to the state where all can appreciate that death is inevitable.

Sometimes there is disagreement about whether death is near. Typically we see this in protracted hospital admissions where the prognosis is less than clear and where there is a long and complex narrative with ample opportunity for miscommunication and even conflict. In our study, this phenomenon was represented in patients whose length of stay exceeded three weeks.

In these patients, we found an *inversion of the usual process of end of life decision making* that was just described. Instead of the more normative sequence of the completion of a DNR order followed by being identified as dying and then being designated for comfort care, these patients were identified as dying by staff, *even before the completion of a DNR order*. In these cases, the comment heard on the floors might be, "He's got end-stage renal cell and is septic . . . and he's not even DNR yet."

The comment captures the essence of a futility dispute where the practitioner feels that disproportionate "curative" interventions are being applied to an incurable patient and that the dying process is being prolonged with its attendant suffering.[33,34] These cases can be powerful experiences and are remembered long after they are over.

In futility disputes, there is discordance between the clinician's sense of where the case is going and the expectations of the patient or family.[35] To the clinician, the patient is dying. But the family has not even taken the first step towards letting go with a DNR order.

This departure from the usual progression of decision making may reflect ambivalence about the "right thing to do" or stem from distrust of the information that is being provided by the clinical team. An especially difficult dynamic can arise when the family believes that the patient's dire condition was precipitated by a medical error or if they are suspicious that substandard care is being provided because the patient is from a traditionally marginalized population.[36,37] In these situations, families will maintain their prerogative to demand care to attempt to right a perceived wrong.

Efforts to mediate such disputes are complicated by preexisting events, perceptions, and distrust.[38] Before we attempt to dissect a futility dispute and understand how they develop and might be prevented, we need to digress and try to define exactly what futility is.

Futility: A Definitional Primer

Although clinicians will often say that they can recognize futility when they see it, the scholarly literature on this topic is broad.[39] There are a number of definitions defining medical futility in the medical ethics literature and some important prerogatives in the law for clinicians to invoke medical futility to withhold and withdraw life-sustaining therapies.[33]

To begin, etymologically, the word futility comes from the Latin *futilis* or leaky. The image is of a vase or container that is unable to hold fluid poured into it. It is a leaky sieve and incapable of producing the desired result, in this case, the storage of fluid.[40] This is actually a helpful image if we consider how often we infuse septic patients with fluids and pressors to *hold* a blood pressure only to see our efforts fail in the face of futile circumstances. In such cases, our efforts are *physiologically futile.*[41]

An intervention is physiologically futile when it can not be performed or is predicted to be unsuccessful with a high degree of medical certainty. An example might be intubation in a patient with an obstructing tracheal mass. Intubation is physiologically futile because the obstruction in the airway cannot be bypassed. Another example might be cardio-pulmonary resuscitation in a patient with an underlying cardiomyopathy who has had recurrent cardiac arrests after multiple resuscitative efforts. Resuscitation in this case is also physiologically futile because the underlying heart disease makes sustained resuscitation impossible. That is, resuscitation is futile because there is nothing that can be done to reverse the underlying myopathy.

The most dramatic invocation of the principle of medical futility is in the setting of a cardiac arrest when the physician in charge determines to "call the code" and acknowledge that his efforts have been unsuccessful. If one can not get a rhythm or bring the pH up to normal range, the likelihood of a successful resuscitation becomes vanishingly smaller and smaller. At that point, the physician invokes the principle of medical futility as ethical justification to stop the resuscitation.

It is important to appreciate that the physiologic definition is the narrowest definition of medical futility. It is a clinical determination based on narrow physiologic parameters. As such it is the definition least open to value judgments about quality of life. For example, although many might feel that it might be futile to treat urosepsis in a patient with advanced Alzheimer's Disease requiring nursing home care, this would not be physiologically futile if there were antibiotics which were effective against the offending bacteria. A physiologic definition simply asks whether the infection could be resolved with antibiotics. If so, the treatment is not physiologically futile, even though the "restoration" of health will be to a pre-morbid state of severe cognitive impairment.

Because the physiologic definition of futility is so narrow—and least open to interpretation—it has been the basis for delineating physician discretion in determining what might constitute futile care.[42] But the narrowness of the physiologic definition is also its greatest weakness and some commentators have offered quantitative and qualitative definitions of medical futility.[43,44] Under the quantitative definition, an intervention is futile if it has not worked in the last one hundred cases. By asserting inefficacy in the prior 100 cases, one exceeds the 95 percent confidence interval used in medicine for other probabilistic decisions. While this definition may be helpful in evaluating isolated technologies, its applicability in the clinical setting is difficult because every case has its nuance and it is difficult to assemble a collection of 100 similar cases to make such a judgment outside of a more controlled research context.

A more helpful concept is the notion of a qualitative definition of medical futility in which one attempts to distinguish physiologic effects from patient-centered treatment benefits. For example, does a medication that raises an ICU patient's blood pressure result in improved cognition? If it simply *effects* a numerical increase in blood pressure without benefit to the patient as a whole, it is qualitatively futile. By distinguishing effect from benefit, this conception of futility asserts that patients are more than their physiology.

Although many clinicians find these definitions an improvement over the more limited physiologic formulation, some commentators worry that physicians undermine patient autonomy and overstep their expertise when they attempt to decide what constitutes a benefit.[45] They maintain that scientific determinations about futility should not be equated with normative judgments about what counts as a "good."

Such arguments limiting the scope of the physician's discretion are countered by equally forceful claims that clinicians should have a small degree of discretion in determining whether treatment is futile when practitioners and families disagree. Without at least some ability to decide that an intervention is futile, physicians would be forced to provide treatments, which they knew were ineffective or even harmful. This would misrepresent medicine's own internal morality.[46,47]

The Evolution of Futility Disputes

Whatever definition of futility we invoke, a fundamental element of any futility dispute is a disagreement between the parties about what constitutes appropriate care. It is this divergence of opinion, perhaps more than the elusive definition of futility, that concerns us here. That is, how do these discordant views take root? What are the factors that lead the clinician to think that the patient is dying while the family remains adamant about the provision of curative care?

Our research—and experience doing ethics case consultations—have led us to believe that many futility disputes are often a product of miscommunication between doctor, patient, and family. Families who demand care believed by clinicians to be futile are often operating upon different assumptions than practitioners because the clinicians have done an inadequate job of communicating basic information about diagnosis, prognosis, and remaining therapeutic or palliative options.[48]

These errors of omission, on the part of clinicians, can engender false hope and lead to requests for care that seem unreasonable. However, these requests become understandable from the perspective of family members if they have not benefited from appropriate and timely conversation and labor under a misconception about the patient's likelihood of recovery.

Figure 4.1
From, Fins JJ. Principles in Palliative Care: An Overview.
Journal of Respiratory Care 2000; 45(11): 1320–1330.

LESSONS FROM FUTILITY DISPUTES

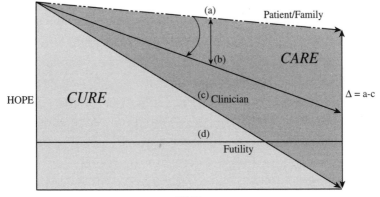

TIME

Let us look at how the expectations of clinicians, patients, and families can diverge, leading to a futility dispute by turning to Figure 4.1.[49] In this graphic, *Hope* is on the Y-axis and *Time* is on the X-axis. At the outset of any illness the course is marked by hopefulness and a commensurate desire for cure.

What this graphic attempts to depict is that the balance of curative and palliative interventions shifts as the trajectory of the illness progresses. In this simplification of a complex dynamic, we see that hope is high at the outset of an illness. If recovery does not occur, hope progressively decreases with new diagnostic or prognostic information or under the weight of burdensome therapy.

This progression affects care strategies and the goals of care, as either primarily curative or palliative.

Unfortunately, in futility disputes the recognition for this change in focus occurs at a different pace for the clinician and the family. This variable awareness of likely outcome is depicted in the differences between *Tanget A*, which represents the hopefulness of patient/family over time, and *Tanget C*, which depicts that of the clinician. Both begin their trajectory at the time of diagnosis but the downward slope (*dh/dt*) is sharper for the clinician than for the patient and family. In most futility disputes, this occurs because the initial hopefulness at the time of diagnosis is not adequately tempered by new knowledge about the patient's deteriorating course. Typically, while the physician gains more knowledge about the progression of disease, this is not communicated to patient and family and their expectations remain higher than might be warranted. Alternatively, information is conveyed but it does not register because of denial or distrust.

Although there is a slight downward inflection to the patient/family curve because they are subjectively aware of some element of decline, it is not as steep as that of the clinician. Over time this leads to a widening gap between the hopes of the patient and family and the clinical realities of the case as perceived by the clinician. This is represented by the delta, $\Delta = A - C$ and illustrates that time is needed for futility disputes to develop because conflicts seldom occur until a dire prognosis becomes evident.

The gap in expectations also has implications for the balance of care and cure. If the patient or family believes that the situation is more hopeful, they will be unprepared to forgo curative interventions and embrace palliation. This discordance between family and clinician can lead to a futility dispute when the gap between *Tangents A* and *C* grows wide or when clinician *Tangent C* bisects a level of hopelessness,

D, which no longer justifies the provision of disproportionate therapies. To return to our study of end-of-life milestones, this would be the dynamic for patients with the long length of stays who are identified as dying by clinicians even before the DNR order is written.

The point that must be stressed when this discordance occurs is that the request for "futile" care may be logical given the information available to the patient or family. Our challenge is to ensure adequate conversation and exchange so that these gaps in understanding are identified early and do not occur. This allows for a more gradual and organic transition from curative interventions to palliative care.

Goal Convergence, Palliative Care, and the Avoidance of Futility Disputes

There is a lot that can be learned from futility disputes about optimizing care near the end of life. A conflict over futility can be thought of as the antithesis of palliative care. Unlike a decision to pursue palliative care or make a referral to hospice where patient, family, and clinicians reach a consensus on the goals of care, futility disputes are marked by conflict and a divergence of perspectives about what is still possible and what is beyond the realm of medical therapy.

When the transition does occur from curative to palliative measures at the end of life, it is emblematic of good communication between the clinician, patient, and family. The discordance of expectations seen in futility disputes is avoided and curative and palliative interventions are balanced, taking note of changes in the patient's course.

Thought of this way, the transition to palliative care becomes simply the exchange of curative goals of care for comfort measures.

Ultimately, the aim should be to reach a mutual understanding about disease trajectory and what goals of care might be appropriate given the changing medical facts and patient/family preferences. We need to be attentive to the pace of these transitions and seek to meet the patient and family halfway as depicted in "consensus," *Tangent B*. By being flexible and appreciating the perspectives of patient and family, we will have an opportunity to achieve a genuine transformation of goals from one dominated by cure to one that is more accepting of care.

These conversations, properly timed and paced, have tremendous potential for improving care. Practically speaking, when clinicians, patients, and families meet routinely to talk about end-of-life care, the benefits can be far greater than expected. These conversations can promote a process of shared decision making, thereby providing an opportunity to develop and enhance the therapeutic relationship. This process builds trust and helps to prevent the widely divergent expectations emblematic of futility disputes.[50]

But as we all know, fostering better communication at the end of life is easier said than done. In the next chapter we will help you build these essential communication skills. We will introduce you to a process of structured goal-setting that promotes a systematic assessment of—and compassionate response to—patient and family needs at the end of life. Through this methodology we hope to provide you with a means to avoid futility disputes and provide palliative care when it is needed most.

References

1 Brock D, Daniel J, and Foley MS. Demography and Epidemiology of Dying in the United States, A Good Dying: Shaping Health Care for the Last Months of Life. Paper Prepared for a Symposium of the *Center to Improve Care of the Dying*, Washington, DC: April 30, 1996.

2 Billings JA and Block S. Palliative Care in Undergraduate Medical Education: Status Report and Future Directions. *Journal of the American Medical Association* 278(9)(1997):733–738.

3 Stevens R. *In Sickness and in Wealth.* New York: Basic Books, 1989.

4 Callahan D. *The Troubled Dream of Life.* New York: Simon and Shuster, 1993.

5 Fins JJ, Miller FG, Acres CA, et al. End-of-Life Decision-Making in the Hospital: Current Practices and Future Prospects. *Journal of Pain and Symptom Management* 17(1)(1999):6–15.

6 Gorowitz S. *Drawing the Line: Life, Death, and Ethical Choices in an American Hospital.* Philadelphia: Temple University Press, 1993.

7 Morrison RS, Ahronheim JC, Morrison GR, et al. Pain and Discomfort Associated with Common Hospital Procedures and Experiences. *Journal of Pain Symptom Management* 15(2)(1998):91–101.

8 Nelson JE, Meier DE, Oei EJ, et al. Self-reported Symptom Experience of Critically Ill Cancer Patients Receiving Intensive Care. *Critical Care Medicine* 29(2)(2001):277–282.

9 Clarke EB, Curtis JB, Luce JM, et al. Robert Wood Johnson Foundation Critical Care End-of-Life Peer Workgroup Members. *Critical Care Medicine* 31(9)(2003):2255–2262.

10 Zussman R. *Intensive Care: Medical Ethics and the Medical Profession.* Chicago: University of Chicago, 1992.

11 I am indebted to anthropologist Sam Beck, Ph.D. for this observation.

12 Fins JJ, Guest RS, and Acres CA. Gaining Insight into the Care of Hospitalized Dying Patients: An Interpretative Narrative Analysis. *Journal of Pain and Symptom Management* 20(6)(2000):399–407.

13 Danis M, Southerland LI, Garrett JM, et al. A Prospective Study of Advance Directives for Life-sustaining Care. *New England Journal of Medicine* 324(13)(1991):882–888.

14 Espinosa E, Gonzalas Baron M, Zamora P, et al. Doctors Also Suffer When Giving Bad News to Cancer Patients. *Supportive Care Cancer* 4(1)(1996):61–63.

15 Youngner S. Do-not-resuscitate Orders: No Longer Secret, but Still a Problem. *Hastings Center Report* 17(1)(1987):24–33.

16 Zussman, *Intensive Care*, 139–160.

17 Danis M, Federman D, Fins JJ, et al. Incorporating Palliative Care into Critical Care Education: Principles, Challenges and Opportunities. *Critical Care Medicine* 27(9)(1999):2005–2013.

18 Wagner GS, Cebe B, and Rozear MP (Eds.). *E.A. Stead, Jr.: What This Patient Needs is a Doctor.* Durham, NC: Carolina Academic Press, 1978.

19 Eachempati SR, Miller FG and Fins JJ. The Surgical Intensivist as Mediator of End-of-Life Issues in the Care of Critically Ill Patients. *Journal of the American College of Surgeons* 197(5)(2003):847–853.

20 Heyland DK, Rocker GM, Dodek PM, et al. Family Satisfaction with Care in the Intensive Care Unit: Results of a Multiple Center Study. *Critical Care Medicine* 30(7)(2002):1413–1418.

21 Fins JJ. Removing the Mask. *The Hastings Center Report* 33(2)(2003):12–13.

22 Fins JJ. Palliation in the Age of Chronic Disease. *The Hastings Center Report* 22(1)(1992):41–42.

23 McClung JA, Kamer RS, DeLuca M, et al. Evaluation of a Medical Ethics Consultation Service: Opinions of Patients and Health Care Providers. *American Journal of Medicine.* 100(1996):456–460.

24 Cassell E. *The Nature of Suffering.* New York: Oxford University Press, 1991.

25 Fins JJ. *Ethics Case Consultation Journals, 1991–Present.* New York: Weill Cornell Medical Center Archives.

26 Fins JJ and Miller FG. Clinical Pragmatism, Ethics Consultation and the Elderly. *Clinics in Geriatric Medicine* 16(1)(2000):71–81.

27 Agrawal SK and Fins JJ. Ethics Committees and Case Consultation in the Hospital Setting. In *A Guide to Hospitals and Inpatient Care.* Siegler E, Mirafzali S and Foust JB, (Eds.) New York: Springer, 2003.

28 Solomon MZ, Jennings BJ, Fins JJ, et al. *Decisions Near the End of Life Faculty Guide*, 3rd ed., Newton, MA: Education Development Center, Inc., 1997.

29 Middlewood S, Gardner G, and Gardner A. Dying in Hospital: Medical Failure or Natural Outcome? *Journal of Pain and Symptom Management* 22(6)(2001):1035–1041.

30 Morrison RS, Meier DE, and Cassel CK. When Too Much is Too Little. *New England Journal of Medicine* 335(23)(1996):1755–1759.

31 Fins JJ. A 38-year-old Man with a Secondary Leukemia who Needs Setting of Goals of Care. In Heffner JE and Byock I (Eds.). *Palliative and End-of-Life Pearls.* Philadelphia: Hanley and Belfus, 2002, pp. 174–176.

32 Solomon MZ, O'Donnell L, Jennings B, et al. Decisions Near the End of Life: Professional Views on Life-Sustaining Treatments. *American Journal of Public Health* 83(1)(1993):14–23.

33 Solomon MZ, Jennings BJ, Crigger BJ, et al. *Futility, Decisions Near the End of Life.* Vol. 7. Newton MA: Education Development Center, 1997.

34 Fins JJ and Solomon MZ. Communication in Intensive Care Settings: The Challenge of Futility Disputes. *Critical Care Medicine* 29(2 Suppl.)(2001):N10–N15.

35 Solomon MZ. How Physicians Talk About Futility: Making Words Mean too Many Things. *Journal of Law, Medicine and Ethics* 21(2)(1993):231–237.

36 Abraham LK. Mama Might Be Better Off Dead. Chicago: The University of Chicago Press, 1993.

37 Crawley LM, Marshall PA, Lo B, et al. End-of-Life Care Consensus Panel. Strategies for Culturally Effective End-of-Life Care. *Annals of Internal Medicine* 136(9)(2002):673–679.

38 Lantos JD. Futility Assessments and the Doctor–Patient Relationship. *Journal of the American Geriatrics Society* 42(8)(1994): 868–870.

39 Fins JJ. Futility in Clinical Practice: Report on a Congress of Clinical Societies. *Journal of the American Geriatrics Society* 42(8)(1994): 861–865.

40 *The Shorter Oxford English Dictionary on Historical Principles.* 3rd Ed. New York: Oxford University Press, 1973.

41 Youngner SJ. Who Defines Futility? *Journal of the American Medical Association* 260(14)(1988):2094–2095.

42 The New York State Task Force on Life and the Law. *When Others Must Choose: Deciding for Patients Without Capacity.* March 1992. Chapter 14.

43 Schneiderman LJ, Jecker NS and Jonsen A. Medical Futility: Its Meaning and Ethical Implications. *Annals of Internal Medicine* 112(2)(1990):949–54.

44 Schneiderman LJ. The Futility Debate: Effective versus Beneficial Intervention. *Journal of the American Geriatrics Society* 42(8)(1994): 883–886.

45 Veatch RM. Why Physicians Cannot Determine if Care is Futile. *Journal of the American Geriatrics Society* 42(8)(1994):871–874.

46 Tomlinson T and Brody H. Futility and the Ethics of Resuscitation. *Journal of the American Medical Association* 264(10)(1990): 1276–1280.

47 Brody H. The Physician's Role in Determining Futility. *Journal of the American Geriatrics Society* 42(8)(1994):875–878.

48 Fins JJ. Breaking the Silence: Futility, Fear and Anger. In *Futility, Decisions Near the End of Life.* Vol. 7. Newton, MA: Education Development Center; 1997:26–27.

49 Fins JJ. Principles in Palliative Care: An Overview. *Journal of Respiratory Care* 45(11)(2000):1320–1330.

50 Dowdy MD, Robertson C, Bander JA. A Study of Proactive Ethics Consultation for Critically and Terminally Ill Patients with Extended Lengths of Stay. *Critical Care Medicine* 26(2)(1998):252–59.

part II

Goal-Setting: A Strategy for Effective Palliative Care

c h a p t e r   f i v e

Goals of Care: Triggering the Process

Goal-Setting as Differential Diagnosis

In this chapter we will introduce you to a process of structured goal setting that will help you provide timely and comprehensive palliative care to dying patients and their families. Goal setting is never futile. It is the way to structure and ensure good communication at the end of life.

Setting goals is both the implicit organizing principle and explicit objectives of end-of-life discussions. A template for this process is the Goals of Care Assessment Tool or GCAT. (See Appendix.) This instrument was a direct outgrowth of our clinical experience with dying patients and our research on practice patterns at the end of life. We designed it to help clinicians engage in a structured process of critical thinking about end-of-life care that would help avoid some of the pitfalls that too often mark life's last chapter.

Using the GCAT as a guide, you will be able to emulate the best practitioners who care for patients at the end of life. While use of the GCAT will not make you more empathic, it will make explicit what skilled practitioners intuitively do for patients near the end of life. It will help you recognize when to introduce a discussion about palliative care and help you become informed about clinical and narrative issues, which should inform the care of each patient and family. So informed, you will be better prepared to formulate a care plan and speak with a patient and family about care options.

The GCAT is comprised of four distinct sections: 1) triggers; 2) collection of clinical and narrative data; 3) formulation of the goals of care; and 4) development of a care plan and consensus building.

This sequence should be familiar to you because it is analogous to the process of differential diagnosis that you employ every day in clinical practice. The *triggers* are like presenting complaints or findings that prompt additional assessment. *Collection of clinical and narrative data* is analogous to doing a history and physical and reviewing laboratory data. Articulating the *goals of care* follows the collection of data just as the construction of a differential diagnosis follows the completion of a history and physical. Like a differential diagnosis, this articulation of the goals of care is an hypothesis that needs to be suggested and confirmed. Using these tentative goals of care, the next step is to suggest a plan of care to patient and family and reach a consensus on next steps.

Just as diagnostic thinking does not guarantee a right answer or correct diagnosis, structured goal setting will not provide you with an answer about what to do. Instead, it will help structure your thinking about cases at the end of life with the same rigor that goes into conventional diagnostic assessment. There may not be a "right" answer about what course to take but there are clinical and narrative elements that *must* be considered before any decision can be made. Anything less informed should be seen as lacking.

We hope that use of the GCAT will help you recognize when you should ask whether the prevailing acute goals of care are applicable and collect the information necessary for effective communication with patients and families about care strategies at the end of life.

Triggering the Process

To improve palliative and end-of-life care, you must first recognize that the patient is dying. These triggers are analogous to presenting symptoms that you routinely encounter when you work up patients. With your training, you have come to recognize what sort of complaint or physical finding should prompt more comprehensive assessment and careful follow-up. We all know that a chronic tension headache is different from one that is also marked by a stiff neck, photophobia and a peticheal rash. The latter should quickly suggest meningiococcal meningitis, an emergency requiring immediate antibiotics and lumbar puncture.

There are similar red flags at the end of life that should trigger a change in course from a curative approach to one that is more directed to pain and symptom management. This is the hardest step in the entire process because we are so heavily acculturated to deny the dying process and so invested in our curative technologies. At this juncture, most of our errors are ones of omission, in which we fail to recognize problematic situations near the end of life that should prompt us to think differently about the care provided.

Unlike the patient presenting with meningitis, the triggers that should prompt a reevaluation of the goals of care can be very subtle. They might be a statement on rounds about "another round of antibiotics," discomfort on a family member's face, or an oblique question from the patient about the future. At other times, it may be the presence of anxiety or tension on a previously well-functioning clinical team.

Too often these sentiments go unexplored and unexamined to the detriment of patient care and the goals of care. It is important to stop and think about these problematic situations and allow your moral intuitions to surface so that they can be made explicit and addressed.[1,2] The best clinicians recognize the subtle signs of disease before they become apparent. With early treatment, lives are saved and morbidity reduced. Similarly, early recognition that death may be near affords patients and families an opportunity to make the most of the time that is remaining and minimize the burden of interventions which are unlikely to extend life.

The eight most common triggers that should prompt a further assessment of the goals of care are identified in Figure 5-1. Each trigger is a milestone—of the sort we discussed in the previous chapter—that calls out for us to take notice and ensure that the current course of care remains appropriate to evolving circumstances.

The triggers are organized under three overarching rubrics when: *the patient is perceived as dying*; *end-of-life decisions are made*; and there is a *significant clinical development*. (See Figure 5-1.) In each section we may digress to

Figure 5-1   Triggers Completion of GCAT

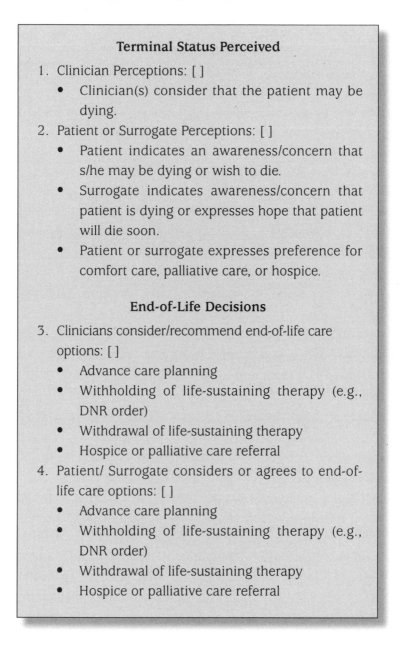

Terminal Status Perceived

1. Clinician Perceptions: [ ]
   * Clinician(s) consider that the patient may be dying.
2. Patient or Surrogate Perceptions: [ ]
   * Patient indicates an awareness/concern that s/he may be dying or wish to die.
   * Surrogate indicates awareness/concern that patient is dying or expresses hope that patient will die soon.
   * Patient or surrogate expresses preference for comfort care, palliative care, or hospice.

End-of-Life Decisions

3. Clinicians consider/recommend end-of-life care options: [ ]
   * Advance care planning
   * Withholding of life-sustaining therapy (e.g., DNR order)
   * Withdrawal of life-sustaining therapy
   * Hospice or palliative care referral
4. Patient/ Surrogate considers or agrees to end-of-life care options: [ ]
   * Advance care planning
   * Withholding of life-sustaining therapy (e.g., DNR order)
   * Withdrawal of life-sustaining therapy
   * Hospice or palliative care referral

Figure 5-1   (continued)

Medical Developments

5. New Diagnostic or Prognostic Information: [ ]
   - Diagnosis of life-threatening illness.
   - Prognosis of < 6 months life expectancy.
6. Change in Clinical Course in Patient With Life-Threatening Illness: [ ]
   - Acute decompensation: e.g., respiratory failure, sepsis, shock, significant change in mental status.
   - Need for life-sustaining therapy: e.g., pressors, ventilator, tube feeding, dialysis.
7. Admission/Transfer to ICU: [ ]
   - Goals should be reassessed upon consideration of ICU Admission.
8. Refractory End-of-Life Symptoms: [ ]
   - Unrelieved distress from pain, dyspnea, anxiety, depression, nausea/vomiting or constipation.

provide you with more information as to how to respond to one of these triggers and place them into context.

Although these triggers are presented sequentially in the next three chapters, this is not meant to imply that this is the order in which they occur. Each trigger can occur alone or in tandem with other developments. And to complicate matters further, different individuals may perceive the patient's course differently. A clinician may interpret new diagnostic information as a harbinger of a terminal outcome, though the patient may be in denial.

Concluding Comments

The 20th Century Spanish philosopher Jose Ortega y Gassett once wrote that we see the world with a repertoire of ideas inside of ourselves and that we need to move beyond our own blindness to see things in a more subtle vein. Or to put it more colloquially, he asserted, that the un-educated eye does not see.[3]

This detailed discussion of triggers is intended to help you better *see* those critical junctures in patient care when it is necessary to reassess the goals of care. Following Ortega y Gasset's admonition, we hope the structure we provide will *educate your eyes to see* more fully all the variables that can inform medical practice at the end of life.

The message is a simple one: good end-of-life care is essentially about observation, picking up clinical and narrative clues that suggest a transition from curative to palliative care. But this is easier said than done. Developing these skills will indeed take time, but it always has. Your challenge today is no different than that articulated by Sir William Osler in his essay, *The Hospital as College* first delivered at The New York Academy of Medicine in 1903:

> The whole art of medicine is in observation, as the old motto goes, but to educate the eye to see, the ear to hear and the finger to feel takes time, and to make a beginning, to start a man on the right track is all we can do. We expect too much of the student and we try to teach him too much. Give him good methods and a proper point of view and all other things will be added as his experience grows.[4]

So do not be overwhelmed by the challenge ahead of you, lest you walk away from your obligations in frustration. The next chapters will give you good methods and a proper point of view so that you will be better able to recognize developments near the end of life and provide better care to your patients.

References

1 Fins JJ, Bacchetta MD, and Miller FG. Clinical Pragmatism: A Method of Moral Problem Solving. *Kennedy Institute of Ethics Journal* 7(2)(1997):129–145.

2 Fins JJ and Miller FG. Clinical Pragmatism, Ethics Consultation and the Elderly. *Clinics in Geriatric Medicine* 16(1)(2000):71–81.

3 Ortega y Gassett J. La Rebelion de Las Masas. In *Jose Ortega y Gasset Obras Completas*, Tomo 4. Madrid: Alianza Editorial, 1983: 186–187.

4 Osler W. The Hospital as a College. In *Aequamimitas*, 1st ed. London: H.K. Lewis, 1904: 327–342.

c h a p t e r   s i x

Goals of Care: When Death Is Near

Introduction

In this chapter we will consider how we recognize when death may be near by focusing on your perceptions as a clinician and those of the patient and family. We will consider some of the subtle signs that will help you recognize distress and the need to reevaluate the goals of care.

Clinical Perceptions

A logical first trigger are your own thoughts. (See Figure 6.1.) Don't discount your intuitions. That *sense* that a patient may be dying is an important one to acknowledge and share with

Figure 6-1 Terminal Status Perceived

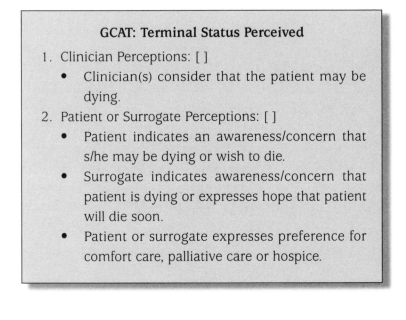

GCAT: Terminal Status Perceived

1. Clinician Perceptions: [ ]
   - Clinician(s) consider that the patient may be dying.
2. Patient or Surrogate Perceptions: [ ]
   - Patient indicates an awareness/concern that s/he may be dying or wish to die.
   - Surrogate indicates awareness/concern that patient is dying or expresses hope that patient will die soon.
   - Patient or surrogate expresses preference for comfort care, palliative care or hospice.

your colleagues. You may be wrong, but it is still important to give voice to your thoughts. Even experienced clinicians have a difficult time prognosticating when death will occur. (The issue of prognostication will be considered later on in our consideration of the GCAT.)

What is important is to stress that you need to be sensitive to your own observations and growing clinical sensibility and raise the question with your colleagues and supervisors. Making intuitions apparent is crucial to improving end-of-life care. Thoughts and perceptions are of no value to the patient or team unless they are articulated and made transparent.

Often times the only thing that will prompt a comment will be the sense that *something* has changed. It may be a change in skin color, diminished appetite, fatigue, dyspnea or a change in affect; changes that occur before lab results portend a decline. You may wonder why aggressive interventions continue when a terminally-ill patient appears to be suffering.

Because you spend so much time with patients, you may be the first to sense a change in course. Much has been written about this phenomenon, particularly in nurses.[1] Nurses and house officers are often the first to sense that the patient is dying. They have more direct patient contact and thus may be the first to pick up on subtle signs that foretell a treatment failure.

Although you and your nursing colleagues may sense that a patient is dying, you often have difficulty articulating why you feel that way. Or you may ask whether you have a right to speak up and voice an "unschooled" opinion. As a result, you may be reluctant to share your perceptions with colleagues, particularly if the attending physician continues to provide aggressive and curative therapies. Issues of power and hierarchy can act as constraints, or the momentum may carry the conversation elsewhere. For the patient's sake, these perceptions should be brought forward.

Your intuitions may be proven incorrect, just as a diagnosis may be proven incorrect when you engage in the process of formulating a differential diagnosis. But like the formulation of a differential diagnosis, the articulation of goals remains valuable regardless of the ultimate conclusion. The purpose of letting your intuitions prompt this process of inquiry is to help ensure that the goals of care remain appropriate to evolving circumstances. In this way, you will help to avoid the errors of omission that too often mark end-of-life care.

Patient Perceptions

Like you, patients and families may sense that death is near. Any indication that the patient knows or suspects that he is dying should prompt a process of structured goal setting. You need to be acutely sensitive to cues that the patient is thinking about death. For instance, the patient may sense that he/she is dying and be suffering emotionally. He may worry about how and when it will happen, how loved ones will cope or if there will be too much pain.

This distress is more about *suffering* than about pain. Clinicians must remember, as Eric Cassell has eloquently noted, that suffering is a subjective state of distress experienced by patients who perceive their fundamental personhood to be threatened or disrupted.[2,3] Fears about mortality, or a death anxiety, even if prospects of death are remote, can engender a substantial existential threat to the self. You can help ameliorate this distress with empathic conversation and therapeutic engagement.

Most of us are aware of those conspiracies of silence that occur in the clinical setting. No one has had a frank conversation with a patient who is dying although all acknowledge that "she knows she is dying." How lonely and afraid she must feel, yet no one intercedes. The belief that she knows she may be dying is used as a self-serving excuse to avoid what could be an uncomfortable situation, for you and the patient.

How would you respond to the patient who asks, "Am I dying?" or says, "I can't take this anymore, I'd rather die than suffer like this." The easiest way to respond might be with a casual or reassuring comment intended to be positive and supportive, but this truncates the conversation and dismisses the patient's need to communicate. Although it is appropriate to defer any major decisions about care to the attending physician, it is important for you to listen to the patient and allow her to voice her concerns.

In talking with the patient, the use of open-ended questions is helpful. You can ask what she thinks is happening with her care and indirectly inquire about her understanding of her disease and prognosis. While you collect important information you can also assure the patient that you will also communicate what you have learned to your attending physician. This approach allows for a timely response to patient needs and indicates that you value what she has told you. It will also establish trust between you and the patient. This is an essential ingredient of any decision-making process.

Many patients are preoccupied by the prospect of their own death but are afraid to broach the issue. There are as many reasons for this as there are fearful patients. Their hesitancy might reflect a cultural reluctance to talk about death and dying or may be for more personal reasons.[4] They may want to remain stoical in front of their doctors, to be "tough," to "fight" and to not "lose hope."[5] They may feel that they risk abandonment if their doctor perceives they are no longer in the fight for a full recovery.[6] More likely than not, patients may not want to confront the truth about their diagnosis or prognosis.

The relationship between doctors and dying patients can further add to these conspiracies of silence. All of us want to be successful as clinicians. When patients we have cared for do not do well, we blame ourselves. At some level we view death as a medical failure,[7] even though we might rationally acknowledge that we did all that was humanly possible. At times we seek shelter in technical language and talk about the details of medical management—the mix of antibiotics, lab results, information on the monitors, or ventilator settings—instead of talking about the big picture.[8] This reluctance to talk frankly about an impending death is often silently communicated to patients, putting this topic off-limits.

For all these reasons, conversations about death and dying may not occur. Patients may be unable—or unwilling—to initiate the conversation because of their own fears, their sense that the doctor is afraid of the topic, or because they fear that they will not encounter a receptive ear from their doctor. Because of this, some patients may be more comfortable initiating this conversation with another member of the health care team, with whom they spend more time or feel more at ease. For example, they may speak openly about the issue with you or a nurse but never mention it to the attending physician. The patient may introduce the topic—and assess your willingness to engage in the conversation—by testing the waters. They may hint about concerns, make a casual comment or even engage in gallows humor. Because we can not know in advance who will become a trusted confidant, every member of the treatment team must watch closely for these signs and *not assume* that someone else has had this important discussion.

When a Patient Wants to Die

Some patients express their thoughts about death by openly communicating a wish to die. The first thing one should do when this occurs is to clarify what they are requesting and not make a hasty decision about care.[9] A desire for death may seem to indicate a request for physician-assisted suicide but usually it indicates that the patient wants to forgo curative care or have life-sustaining therapy withdrawn. So when a patient indicates a wish to die, we must avoid jumping to conclusions and better define the request. Furthermore, it is important to understand that this wish may be the consequence of treatable distress.

An expressed desire to die may be a sign of a depression or part of the patient's coping mechanisms.[10] Many studies have investigated terminal patients' desire to die in relation to requests of physician-assisted suicide. While some patients cited the physical distress of pain and other symptoms as their primary reason to seek death, the characteristic that distinguished these patients from those who did not express these things was a pervasive sense of hopelessness.[11]

Hopelessness and a desire for death are primary symptoms of depression, which is quite common among the terminally ill. Nonetheless, depression is *not* normative in terminal illness. It is clinically inappropriate to "write off" a dying patient's depression as simply something that goes along with their terminal illness. Depression can and should be treated in patients in all phases of the life cycle, including those at the end of life.

It is striking to note that an estimated 25 percent of patients with advanced cancer suffer from depression at some time and that over 80 percent of these patients are never treated. Diagnosing depression in these patients is complicated by the false assumption that depression is expected in this setting and by the shared symptomatology of advanced cancer and depression: weight loss, fatigue, and hypersomnia. These physical findings mimic many of the classic symptoms of depression. In addition to depression, a wish to die has been correlated with poor pain management, lack of social support, and other issues possibly amenable to medical, social, or psychiatric interventions.[12,13,14,15,16]

If it is determined that a patient is making a request for assisted suicide, you need to be careful not to be prejudicial about the request.[17] While you will never be obliged to assist a patient with a suicide—and, as of publication of this text, such assistance is illegal in all states but Oregon at the time of the publication of this text—you have an affirmative obligation to explore a patient's request fully and comprehensively without being judgmental.[18] It is important to maintain *clinical neutrality* in order to understand the patient's motivations and fears.

If you come to these discussions convinced that assisted suicide is morally wrong, you run the risk of adding guilt to the patient's distress. Patients make such requests of clinicians whom they trust and with great trepidation and are reflective of physical, psychological, or existential distress.

Because of these factors, you need to be careful not to be moralistic. Patients have come to you in need of help. Your response should not undermine the trust they have placed in you but rather bolster the doctor–patient relationship, which itself can be therapeutic. Conversely, if you are ideologically predisposed to assisted suicide, it is critical that you maintain neutrality lest you be too permissive in acquiescing to a request.[19]

Maintaining this balance may be difficult because you will likely already have an opinion on this issue. It has been shown that a physician's receptivity to a request for assisted suicide correlates with his religious beliefs as well as other demograghic considerations such as medical specialty, age, and practice setting.[20,21]

If you understand the patient's motivations, there may be other ways to address these concerns. For example, a patient may worry about "being a burden on his family" or "dying in the hospital, in pain." A request may be motivated by fear and in response to a new diagnosis or prognostic information. Each of these scenarios will suggest different therapeutic responses. But you will only be able to help if these concerns are brought to light and if further conversation is facilitated.

Whether it is in response to an explicit request for assisted suicide or a side-long glance that indicates fear, the doctor–patient relationship is most therapeutic when you answer questions, provide psychological support, and manage the patient's symptom burden. These encounters will be professionally rewarding, providing an unparallel opportunity to gain insight into a patient's beliefs, values, and wishes and to *recognize the person in the patient.*

Surrogate Perceptions

It is not surprising that family members might be the first to sense that something is not right and believe that a patient may be dying. They have seen the patient's response to treatment, good and bad, and recognize a downward course. Significant others know who the patient was *before the disease took over.* They have more perspective because they can see what is happening in light of the patient's life narrative. This shared past, with its deep bonds and intimate knowledge, makes family members natural advocates for the patient. So, just as the patient's questions and comments should trigger inquiry and assessment, so too should the impressions of family members and close friends.

Each of us needs to be sensitive to the hidden meaning of comments made by the family and friends of a terminally-ill patient. Expressions of guilt, sadness, and frustration may be clues that loved ones perceive the patient to be suffering or that they believe that the treatments are futile.

The daughter of a patient on a ventilator may say to a nurse, " I hope that Dad passes on soon. I hate to see him suffer like this." This comment suggests that the current level of care and the family's goals are incongruent. Sometimes, the voicing of concern can be more subtle. Indeed a seemingly innocent question asking how much longer a patient needs to be on a ventilator may implicitly be asking whether it need be continued. Whether these concerns are explicitly raised or not, we need to be attentive to what is being implied.

However, when sharing information with family and friends, we need to know at what point we turn to a surrogate in lieu of the patient. If we direct our conversations to the surrogate while the patient is still able to participate in these discussions, we deprive the patient of her right to make medical decisions. This becomes ethically problematic if we take self-determination and the doctrine of informed consent seriously. As noted in Part I, each adult patient has a right to direct our medical care, unless decision-making capacity is lost or a decision has been made not to exercise one's self-determination and cede one's autonomy to another. And these rights extend to decisions at the end of life.[22] To know when the locus of decision making shifts from the patient to a surrogate, we need to briefly digress and consider decision-making capacity.

Decision-Making Capacity

The concept of decision-making capacity is central to the determination of whether decision-making authority resides with the patient or with a surrogate, a substitute decision maker. Adult patients are presumed to have capacity to make medical decisions. When this ability is questioned, capacity can be formally assessed.[23] This is a clinical determination. A determination of capacity hinges on the patient being able to satisfy four requirements. The patient must be able to: (1) understand proposed treatment or care options; (2) apply that information to the particular context; (3) consider the decision in light of personal beliefs and values and; (4) to clearly communicate these choices.[24]

The most widely used standard for assessing capacity focuses on the patient's functional ability to make decisions.[25] We present here a definition, which combines the terminology and elements of the President's Commission for the Study of Ethical Problems in Medicine and Biomedical and Behavioral Research, and the scholarship of Applebaum and Grisso.[26,27] Using this framework, capacity can be defined as the patient's ability to do the following:

- *Understand relevant information.* This may be affected by the patient's attention span, memory deficits, or intelligence.
- *Communicate with others about the information presented.* The patient must be able to respond and explain his/her choices. Level of consciousness, thought disorders, short-term memory problems or ambiguity may interfere with this ability.
- *Appreciate the situation and its consequences.* The patient must be able to explain his/her illness, the need for treatment, and what could be expected to happen with or without treatment. Denial and delusion could affect this ability.
- *Reason about the choices in terms of personal goals and values.* Patients should be able to explain their decisions. Psychosis, dementia, delirium, phobias, and anger may interfere.

Generally we speak of a patient satisfying a rational standard for making decisions, that is, there is evidence that the patient is thinking about his or her choices with a degree of logic and coherence. Psychosis, dementia, delirium, phobias, and anger may interfere with the patient's ability to make a rational assessment. Some commentators also assert that the degree of coherence and understanding demonstrated by a patient should be commensurate with the seriousness of the decision that is being considered.[28] For example, a decision to refuse a trivial or elective procedure would require less justification than refusal of one that might be lifesaving.

It is important to note that a patient's capacity is *specific* to the question being asked and *not* a global determination of cognitive abilities. Patients can retain decision-making capacity, even if they have an element of cognitive impairment, so long as it does not compromise their ability to understand treatment choices.

In addition, in the clinical context, capacity can wax and wane. Because patients can gain and lose capacity as their medical condition changes, it is important to remain attentive to changes in mental status that may have a bearing on the patients ability to participate in decision making.

Some cases of decisional incapacity may be reversible, such as delirium from hypercalcemia. Whenever possible, reversible cause of incapacity should be treated to vest authority with the patient, unless treatment is associated with disproportionate burdens. (For example, it would be ethically inappropriate to reverse analgesia needed for intractable pain to ask a patient about their preferences.)

In most cases, it is clear when authority for medical decisions should be assumed by a surrogate. When it is not, as in the case when a patient asserts his or her right to make a decision, which seems to indicate a lack of judgment, clinicians can turn to the court for guidance. A judge can hear the evidence about the patient's ability to make the decision in question and determine whether the patient should retain that right or find that the patient is incompetent and that a surrogate must decide what should be done. It is important to appreciate that capacity is a clinical judgment, while the determination of *competence*, with its implications for civil liberties, is a judicial ruling.

Helping Surrogates Decide

Although the courts are available to adjudicate disputes, the vast majority of surrogates assume authority for making decisions without conflict. They step in when patients have lost their ability to make independent judgments. Nonetheless, surrogates need direction in how to exercise their authority.

It is generally accepted that surrogates should be guided in their decisions by the patient's previously articulated preferences or *expressed wishes* if they are known.[29] If specific knowledge of patient wishes is lacking, then the surrogate should invoke *substituted judgment*. When substituted judgment is invoked, decisions are informed by what the surrogate believes the patient would have done in the given circumstances. Here the surrogate is asked to make judgments with the patient's values and life experiences in mind. The last category is called the *best interests* standard. In the absence of information to guide substituted judgment, surrogates together with clinicians, should determine a plan of care that promotes the patient's best interests in light of the benefits and burdens of treatment options. This is a generic standard used when nothing about the preferences of a particular patient are known. Here the issue is what sort of decision a reasonable person would make, balancing benefits and burdens.[30,31]

When confronted with a decision, the surrogate should use an understanding of the patient's beliefs and feelings in order to reach the same conclusion the patient would have reached had he/she been able.[32] Several studies have attempted to measure the accuracy of decisions made by surrogates, finding that surrogate choices are in line with those of the patient 57–81 percent of the time and that these rates may improve if patients discussed their views on end-of-life care with their surrogates directly.[33,34,35] (For more information on the surrogate's role in advance directives, see page 125–132.)

In addition to determining how decisions should be made, it is also critical to determine who has *priority among potential surrogates*.[36] Although the decision-making hierarchy can differ from state to state, some general rules apply.[37] The surrogate with the highest standing is one deliberately chosen by the patient while they still had decision-making capacity utilizing an advance directive (see below).[38] A designated surrogate has standing because his or her authority originates directly from the patient's exercise of autonomy. Depending upon jurisdiction, a designated surrogate is known as a durable power of attorney for healthcare, a health care agent, or more colloquially a health care proxy. (For the purposes of this volume we will refer to a designated surrogate as a proxy.)

If the patient did not designate a proxy, we turn to the next of kin generally in this order: spouse, adult child, parent, adult sibling, close friend. A court-appointed guardian could supersede the authority of family members. The authority of a proxy chosen by the patient while still competent, however, has been viewed as being protected from judicial trumping.[39]

Some states also permit close friends to step in as a surrogate, if there is no available blood relative. In some cases, individuals in this category are in a committed relationship with the patient. Although they have standing in some jurisdictions, they are vulnerable to being trumped by someone who is higher on the list who is *biologically* related. These issues are particularly timely as our nation debates the question of gay marriage. Proponents of gay marriage assert that the partner of a patient should have higher standing than a biological relative when a significant other is hospitalized.[40] Until we reach a societal consensus on the broader question of gay marriage, it seems prudent to counsel an unmarried patient with a significant other to designate their partner as their proxy to ensure that their wishes will be articulated by a trusted intimate.[41]

Surrogates play a large role in palliative care because many patients lose decision-making capacity at the very end of life and can not participate in difficult choices. This can place a tremendous moral and psychological burden on surrogates. In order to ease this burden as well as respect self-determination, practitioners should encourage patients to engage in *advance care planning* by discussing their preferences with their loved ones while they are still able to communicate with them. Advance care planning is discussed in the next chapter.

References

1 Baggs JG and Schmitt MH. End-of-life Decisions in Adult Intensive Care: Current Research Base and Directions for the Future. *Nursing Outlook* 48(4)(2000):158–164.
2 Cassell EJ. The Nature of Suffering and the Goals of Medicine. *New England Journal of Medicine* 306(1982):639–645.
3 Cassell EJ. *The Nature of Suffering and the Goals of Medicine.* New York: Oxford University Press, 1991.

4 Blackhall LJ, Frank G, Murphy S, et al. Bioethics in a Different Tongue: The Case of Truth-telling. *Journal of Urban Health* 78(1)(2001): 59–71.

5 Fins JJ. The Inner Life of a Stoic Facing Death. A Review of 'Cancer: A Personal Voyage.' *Journal of Pain and Symptom Management* 15(3)(1998):208–209.

6 Weinman Lear M. *Heart Sounds.* New York: Random House Value Publishing, 1988.

7 Wanzer SH, Adelstein SJ, Cranford RE, et al. The Physician's Responsibility Toward Hopelessly Ill Patients. *New England Journal of Medicine* 310(15)(1984):955–999.

8 Zussman R. *Intensive Care: Medical Ethics and the Medical Profession.* Chicago: University of Chicago, 1992.

9 Bascom PB and Tolle SW. Responding to Requests for Physician-Assisted Suicide: 'These are uncharted waters for both of us . . .' *Journal of the American Medical Association* 288(1)(2002):91–98.

10 Van Loon RA. Desire to Die in Terminally Ill People: A Framework for Assessment and Intervention. *Health and Social Work* 24(4)(1999):260–268.

11 Wilson KG, Scott JF, Graham ID, et al. Attitudes of Terminally Ill Patients Toward Euthanasia and Physician-Assisted Suicide. *Archives of Internal Medicine* 160(16)(2000):2454–2460.

12 Lloyd-Williams M. "Difficulties in Diagnosing and Treating Depression in the Terminally Ill Cancer Patient." *Postgraduate Medicine,* 76(899)(2000):555–558.

13 Chochinov HM, Wilson KG, Enns M, et al. Desire for Death in the Terminally Ill. *American Journal of Psychiatry* 152(8)(1995):1185–1191.

14 Cohen LM, Steinberg MD, Hails KC, et al. Psychiatric Evaluation of Death-Hastening Requests: Lessons from Dialysis Discontinuation. *Psychosomatics* 41(3)(2000):195–203.

15 Sachs GA, Ahronheim JC, Rhymes JA, et al. Good Care of Dying Patients: The Alternative to Physician-assisted Suicide and Euthanasia. *Journal of American Geriatric Society* 43(5)(1995): 553–562.

16 Muskin PR. The Request to Die: Role for a Psychodynamic Perspective on Physician-assisted Suicide. *Journal of the American Medical Association* 279(4)(1998):323–328.

17 Fins JJ. Physician Assisted Suicide and the Right to Care. *Cancer Control: Journal of the Moffitt Cancer Center* 3(3)(1996):272–278.

18 Tulsky JA, Ciampa R and Rosen EJ. Responding to Legal Requests for Physician-Assisted Suicide. *Annals of Internal Medicine* 312(6)(2000): 494–499.

19 Quill TE. Death and Dignity: A Case of Individualized Decision Making. *New England Journal of Medicine* 324(10)(1991):691–694.

20 Cohen JS, Fihn SD, Boyko EJ, et al. Attitudes Towards Assisted Suicide and Euthanasia among Physicians in Washington State. *New England Journal of Medicine* 331(2)(1994):89–94.

21 Bachman JG, Alcser KH, and Doukas DJ. Attitudes of Michigan Physicians and the Public toward Legalizing Physician-assisted Suicide and Voluntary Euthanasia. *New England Journal of Medicine* 334(5)(1996): 303–309.

22 Welie JV and Welie SP. Patient Decision Making Competence: Outlines of a Conceptual Analysis. *Medicine, Health Care and Philosophy* 4(2)(2001):127–138.

23 Zaubler TS, Viederman M, and Fins JJ. Ethical, Legal, and Psychiatric Issues in Capacity, Competence, and Informed Consent: An Annotated Bibliography of Representative Articles. *General Hospital Psychiatry* 18(3)(1996):155–172.

24 Tunzi M. Can the Patient Decide? Evaluating Patient Capacity in Practice. *American Family Physician*, 64(2)(2001):299–306.

25 President's Commission for the Study of Ethical Problems in Medicine and Biomedical and Behavioral Research. *Making Health Care Decisions*, Vol 1. Washington, DC: US Government Printing Office, 1982.

26 Applebaum PS and Grisso T. Assessing Patients' Capacities to Consent to Treatment. *New England Journal of Medicine* 319(25)(1988): 1635–1638.

27 Fletcher JC, Lombardo PA, Marchall MF, Miller FG. *Introduction to Clinical Ethics.* 2nd ed. Maryland: University Publishing Group, 1997: 73–76.

28 Drane JF. Competency to Give an Informed Consent. A Model for Making Clinical Assessments. *Journal of the American Medical Association* 252(7)(1984):925–927.

29 President's Commission for the Study of Ethical Problems in Medicine and Biomedical and Behavioral Research. *Deciding to Forego Life-Sustaining Therapy.* Washington, DC: US Government Printing Office, 1983.

30 Buchanan AE and Brock DW. *Deciding for Others: The Ethics of Surrogate Decision Making.* New York: Cambridge University Press, 1990: 15–211.

31 Sachs GA and Siegler M. Guidelines for Decision Making when the Patient is Incompetent. *Journal of Critical Care Illness* 6(1991): 348–359.

32 Weile JV. Living Wills and Substituted Judgements: A Critical Analysis. *Medicine, Health Care and Philosophy* 4(2)(2001):169–183.

33 Hare J, Pratt C, and Nelson C. "Agreement Between Patients and Their Self-Selected Surrogates on Difficult Medical Decisions. *Archives of Internal Medicine* 152(5)(1992):1049–1054.

34 Sulmasy DP, Terry PB, Weisman CS, et al. The Accuracy of Substituted Judgements in Patients with Terminal Diagnoses. *Annals of Internal Medicine* 128(8)(1998):621–629.

35 Sulmasy DP, Haller K, and Terry PB. More Talk, Less Paper: Predicting the Accuracy of Substituted Judgements. *The American Journal of Medicine* 96(5)(1994):432–438.

36 Terry PB, Vettese M, Song J, et al. End-of-Life Decision Making: When Patients and Surrogates Disagree. *Journal of Clinical Ethics* 10(4)(1999):286–293.

37 The New York State Task Force on Life and the Law. *When Others Must Choose: Deciding for Patients Without Capacity*. New York, 1992: 47–69.

38 Brock DW. Trumping Advance Directives. *Hastings Center Report* 21(5)(1991):S5–6.

39 Blake DC, Maldonado L, and Meinhardt RA. *Whittier Law Review* 14(1993):119–44.

40 Clarkson-Freeman PA. The Defense of Marriage Act (DOMA): Its Impact on Those Seeking Same Sex Marriage. *Journal of Homosexuality* 48(2)(2004):1–19.

41 Stein GL and Bonuck KA. Attitudes on End-of-life Care and Advance Care Planning in the Lesbian and Gay Community. *Journal of Palliative Medicine* 4(2)(2001):173–90.

chapter seven

Goals of Care: End-of-Life Decisions

Introduction

There are a number of decision points along an illness trajectory when we should stop and think about goals of care. Whether it is consent to a DNR order, completion of an advance directive in the outpatient setting, or a decision for comfort care, or hospice referral, these occasions provide an opening for discussion.

In this chapter we will discuss DNR orders and advance care planning. We will go into considerable detail and may seem to digress from our discussion of the GCAT and the triggers that should prompt goal setting. A detailed discussion

Figure 7-1 End-of-Life Decisions

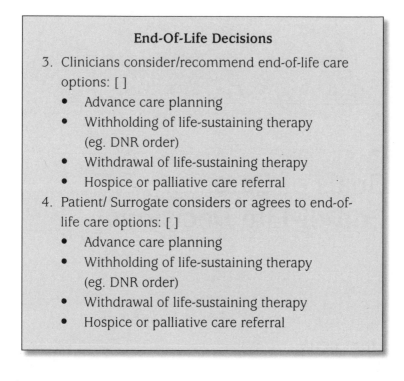

End-Of-Life Decisions

3. Clinicians consider/recommend end-of-life care options: [ ]
   • Advance care planning
   • Withholding of life-sustaining therapy (eg. DNR order)
   • Withdrawal of life-sustaining therapy
   • Hospice or palliative care referral
4. Patient/ Surrogate considers or agrees to end-of-life care options: [ ]
   • Advance care planning
   • Withholding of life-sustaining therapy (eg. DNR order)
   • Withdrawal of life-sustaining therapy
   • Hospice or palliative care referral

about DNR orders, advance directives, and decisions to withdraw life-sustaining therapy and hospice referral is critically important. These designations can often dictate the way care is given and received and choices are conveyed. If we might offer a metaphor, these legal terms are to end-of-life care what grammar and syntax is to language. Without an understanding of these underlying rules, it becomes difficult to appreciate the meaning and content of our discourse at the end of life.

You need to understand these milestones in order to make patients and their loved ones more aware of their treatment options.[1,2] One survey of a large group of outpatients in an Oregon university hospital network revealed wide-spread misunderstanding of choices surrounding end-of-life care.[3] Discussions among the physician, patient, and patient's family about a patient's preferences for end-of-life care can clarify misunderstandings and begin to define goals of care for the patient.

Do Not Resuscitate Orders

A patient or surrogate who consents to a do-not-resuscitate order (DNR) refuses resuscitation in the event of a cardio-pulmonary arrest. In the hospital setting, resuscitation is considered to be the provision of advanced cardiac life support. DNR orders only pertain to care provided in the setting of an arrest and patients with a DNR order are not precluded from the provision of ICU care or surgical interventions which may help achieve palliative goals of care.[4,5]

Many mistake the writing of a DNR order as if it were a comprehensive strategy for palliative care.[6] It is not. A DNR order is simply a plan for the last fifteen minutes of a patient's life. While these orders can help protect a patient from the burdens of an unwanted, and often futile, resuscitative effort, they do little to direct end-of-life care. *The mere absence of resuscitation does not constitute an affirmative plan for pain relief and psychosocial support.*

Too often clinicians attempt to "get a DNR order" or "make a patient DNR," forgetting that patients and surrogates *consent* to this order and are not made to do so. This effort becomes an end in itself and not an opportunity to engage in genuine planning for end-of-life care.

Consider the patient who consents to a DNR order—not to be resuscitated. That designation means that resuscitation will be foregone in the event of a cardiac or respiratory arrest. But what should you do in the six hours before an anticipated arrest as the patient's condition worsens and his pO2 drops and he becomes hypercapneic? Normally, these signs of respiratory failure would lead to intubation. But should a patient who is DNR be intubated to address an impending respiratory arrest? You think not; after all, the patient did consent to a DNR order.

Technically, a DNR designation only takes effect when the patient has stopped breathing or the heart has ceased to beat. So if we strictly construct the law, even patients with a DNR order should be intubated, unless the patient or surrogate said otherwise. And that is the point. A DNR conversation, with a lone focus on resuscitation, is inadequate alone to guide care. Additional questions must be asked. Does the patient want to be intubated? Would he want to go to the intensive care unit if the situation deteriorated? Does the patient want to go to hospice? Unless you ask these questions, a discussion about DNR will lead to the ethical quandary just posed about semi-urgent intubation.

Given these data, your intuition that a patient who has agreed to a DNR order would not want to be intubated may be correct, but you wouldn't know unless you ask. And the DNR discussion may be the last time the patient will be in a position to talk with you before decision-making capacity is lost.

In our experience and the experience of others,[7] patients rarely initiate a discussion about resuscitation. Clinicians need to prompt these conversations. So when DNR is raised by the patient or the family, you need to be particularly sensitive to their distress. Such a request is not normative or common.

It is more common for clinicians to bring up the issue. Generally, it is ethically appropriate to broach a DNR order when the patient's prognosis is grim, the likelihood of a successful resuscitation is low, or when the burden of continued care is high.

In these situations, the clinician should introduce the issue of resuscitation gently with open-ended questions about the patient's knowledge of his situation and about goals and expectations. If this points to an accurate awareness of the situation, you might want to suggest that, "some patients in your condition have developed views on resuscitation and going on a ventilator if their condition deteriorates. Have you ever considered this?"

Sometimes patients and families fear that they will receive less attentive care because they have consented to a DNR order.[8] This fear is not unwarranted because many times house officers and other clinicians will prioritize the needs of other patients over those that are dying, especially if they have a DNR order in place.

Although ethical norms and the law require that care decisions other than resuscitation not be conditioned upon the presence or absence of a DNR order, the completion of a DNR order often heralds a different sort of care. The ICU patient who is made DNR with comfort care is often transferred out of the unit to step-down or a general medical/surgical unit. An attending physician may visit less frequently or delegate responsibility to junior colleagues. The family immediately notices that there is a different level of nursing care and may feel that nobody comes into the room, hence they may experience a sense of abandonment.[9]

There is some basis for this fear of abandonment. Because a DNR order is predicated upon the right to be left alone (see Chapter 3), discussions between physicians, patients, and families often focus on what will *not* be done for the patient, without much, if any, mention of what will and can be done. Lamentably, DNR orders sometimes can become an abbreviation for *do-not-respond*. This only fuels the perception among the laiety that patients with DNR orders will receive less than attentive care. This fear of abandonment is especially prominent amongst some minorities, most notably, African-Americans, who are less likely to consent to a DNR order.[10] It is important to understand why this community is hesitant to embrace decisions to forego life-sustaining therapy and how these views are a microcosm of broader societal issues.[11] Many fear that perceived health care disparities will be compounded if a DNR order is in place.[12–14]

A way to temper the shock that can follow a DNR discussion is to precede it with a discussion about advance care planning; the completion of an advance directive stipulating what the patient would want done if they were so ill they could not speak for themselves. While a DNR conversation asks what should be done if there is a cardio-pulmonary arrest, which is often imminent, engaging in discussions about advance care planning is more about hypothetical and future events. As such, advance care planning can introduce the need to think about end-of-life care and set the stage for subsequent discussions about resuscitation.

The utility of linking DNR orders and advance directive is illustrated nicely if we consider the growing phenomenon of the *partial DNR order* in which the patient consents to some elements of resuscitation but not others.[15] An example might be what is described as a Do Not Intubate or DNI order. In this example a patient might agree to "being shocked" but refuse to be placed on a ventilator. These decisions are generally reflective of patient ambivalence and poorly conceived plans of care. Moreover they place clinicians in an integrity-compromising position because they compel us to offer an incomplete resuscitative intervention that is only marginally effective even when done comprehensively. The data indicate that in-hospital resuscitation results in only 23% survival to discharge, with a range of successful resuscitation varying upon whether the patient had a primary cardiac condition (30%) or end-stage disease (8%).[16]

In the case of the patient who agrees to defibrillation but not ventilation, we might speculate that the patient wants to survive because of agreement to cardioversion, but does not want to linger on a ventilator. The patient is ambivalent about the goals of care and the means to achieve them. A better and more comprehensive approach is to suggest that the patient receive all critical elements of resuscitation and *not* be DNR. This will satisfy the desire for survival. In addition he would be encouraged to complete an advance directive that would provide guidance on his wishes regarding prolonged mechanical ventilation and respect the right to refuse this intervention. By coupling a DNR order with an advance directive, patient wishes can be more accurately achieved and clinical integrity can be preserved. Efforts at resuscitation can then be represented as potentially efficacious and not simply a low utility charade.

Advance Care Planning

Through an advance directive, a patient authorizes a proxy decision maker to make care decisions on her behalf and/or completes a living will, which outlines treatment choices. Advance directives can either be oral statements or written documents and are recognized under state and federal law.[17,18]

A discussion about advance care planning should be the first conversation about care at the end of life between a patient and their physician. Many professional organizations view these discussions as preventive health care and as an important building block of the doctor–patient relationship.[19,20] In this section we will review the types of advance directives used in clinical practice, how to talk with patients and surrogates about advance care planning, and conclude with a discussion of the sort of dilemmas encountered by patients and their proxies.

There are basically three types of advance directives. The first conveys a patient's substantive wishes through a written document called a *living will*. As such, a living will can be considered a treatment directive that lays out the patient's choices regarding therapy. The second type of advance directive gives authority to a chosen surrogate to act on the patient's behalf. This designated surrogate may be known as a *durable power of attorney for health care*, *health care agent*, or even *proxy* depending upon state law and local custom. The third document is a combination of the previous two; a durable power of attorney is appointed by the patient but there is also a section to include additional written instructions.

Whatever the form, an advance directive is a legal document intended to extend the patient's autonomy concerning medical decisions beyond the time when the patient's decision-making capacity is limited or non-existent.[21] Each type has advantages and liabilities.[22,23]

A living will can be helpful when a patient has not identified a designated surrogate to empower as his or her agent. This may be because the patient is isolated and alone or does not feel able to trust another with the responsibilities of surrogacy.

Generally it is better for patients to designate a proxy instead of having a living will if that is an option for them. Living wills have limited utility in the clinical context, although they are better than no advance care planning at all. They may be too vague when describing clinical circumstances, such as when "death is imminent." [24] Living wills can be difficult to interpret because the language is often generic, "If I am ever in a terminal condition, as deemed by my attending physician, I would not want extraordinary measures . . ." Terms like "terminal condition" and "extraordinary measures" are open to interpretation and liable to be informed by the views of the attending physician who is asked to render an opinion.

Or a patient's wishes may be ambiguous, such as a request not to be intubated.[25] This statement may be intended to prevent intubation in the context of a terminal condition, but the patient may feel differently, if a short-term is necessary for recovery. At the other extreme, some living wills may be too specific in their instructions. These instructions may be inapplicable to a patient's situation or so detailed as to completely lose sight of the overriding goals that should guide care.[26]

The lesson here is that when talking with your patients about their treatment choices, it is important to focus on goals and not treatments like intubation. While a statement to forgo intubation may be instructive in a patient who has end-stage COPD and lung cancer and has previously been intubated, it is less helpful in a healthy 40 year old. What does that patient mean? In all likelihood, he wants to avoid being intubated if there is no hope of recovery. He probably does not mean that he would refuse intubation for an emergency splenectomy following a motor vehicle accident.

Finally, because living wills are written documents, they may fail to have the impact of a proxy who can serve as a visible advocate for the patient. Empirical research has shown that a patient's preferences are more likely to be followed if an advance directive has a proxy or durable power of attorney component.[27]

If at all possible, it is advisable that patients complete a healthcare proxy.[28] Designating a proxy is more effective because it empowers a surrogate to make decisions on the patient's behalf and gives the surrogate special legal standing to make a range of end-of-life decisions. Proxies speak for the decisionally incapacitated patient and can agree to treatment, choose between treatment options, refuse or withdraw life-sustaining treatments, ask for better pain management and symptom control, or request a hospice referral. Most importantly, in contrast to a living will, a proxy can apply the patient's values to changing medical circumstances.[29,30]

It is important that patients be helped in choosing appropriate proxies to represent them should they lose decisional capacity. The individual chosen should know the patient's preferences and values and goals. You can help your patients choose a proxy by suggesting that they think of conversations with potential candidates as an *audition* in which the patient determines if the choice of proxy is a good one and the proxy tries on the role as well.[31] Meeting a proxy in the office before he or she assumes these responsibilities can also start a relationship with you before a crisis strikes.

This preparation is critical. Although we speak about advance care planning as an exercise in patient autonomy, it is critically important to appreciate that the designation of a surrogate places a weighty moral responsibility on the proxy as well. This means that the patient has an obligation to be sure that his or her proxy is prepared for this responsibility.[32] You can help foster these conversations by educating patients and their proxies about their *reciprocal obligations* to each other and encourage them to talk about values and preferences in a timely fashion.

Changes in the patient's medical condition or important family events like marriage, divorce, or a new child should also prompt a periodic review of the appropriateness of a proxy and the patient's values.[33] In some states, such personal developments have legal implications with respect to proxy designation.[34] Clinicians should also review the content of advance directives on a yearly basis with their patients to ensure that they remain accurate and timely. In my practice, I couple this review with the yearly effort to inoculate patients against the flu, so as to stay current with regard to patient preferences and choice of proxy.

Working with the Proxy

An advance directive is activated when the patient loses capacity (see prior section). It is important to be attentive to loss of capacity so that an appropriate surrogate can step in to make decisions on behalf of the patient.

Working with the proxy can be rewarding and challenging. It is always better if you begin the doctor–proxy relationship before the patient loses capacity. It might be in the out-patient setting when the advance directive is completed or upon admission when the patient still has capacity.

Either dynamic is better than meeting the surrogate for the first time just after the patient has had an event and lost her ability to communicate. Those occasions are often anxious ones and marked with suspicion. The proxy may be thinking, but not articulating, "What went wrong? Why did this happen to my mother? And who is this doctor, anyway?"

It does not matter that you have cared for the patient for years and that she thought the world of you. Now you have to work with the proxy. It is far better if you have a preexisting relationship of trust. Establishing these relationships prospectively also helps to temper unreasonable and unrealistic demands from a surrogate who is just coming on to the scene.

When working with the proxy, you need to appreciate that this is a time of tremendous stress. The proxy who likely had a long and loving relationship is now being asked to make decisions about the patient without his or her counsel. In a published study that we conducted looking at the patient–proxy relationship, patients and proxies had often known each other for upwards of fifty years.[30]

Although this stress might be mitigated by preparation, it still is critical to recognize and acknowledge the proxy's grief and distress. Although it might seem platitudinous to say: "being a proxy right now must be really difficult, I gather you knew Mrs. Smith for fifty years," respecting the depth of these relationships is very important and potentially therapeutic. Besides, it is the right thing to do.

A particular challenge for the proxy are those situations when they may have difficulty pursuing a choice outlined by the patient. For example, a patient might have asked the proxy to "do everything, no matter what." But now the circumstances have changed. All that is left to offer a patient is a highly burdensome and therapeutically dubious intervention. What should the proxy do? Should she adhere to the patient's prior wish and maintain her fidelity? Or should the proxy demonstrate regard and concern for the patient by forsaking this intervention and protecting the patient from an avoidable harm?

The conventional argument is that the predicate for advance care planning is that the wishes of the patient should be followed and that we should avoid "trumping" an advance directive.[35] If prior wishes are too easily overridden, the integrity of advance care planning will erode and advance directives, as a mechanism for self-determination, will be compromised.

A counter argument, emerging in the bioethics literature,[32,36] is that the patient–proxy relationship is more complex than simply following patient wishes. Defining a proxy as one who is but the sterile conveyor of a patient's prior preferences is to dismiss the deeper ties that often link the patient and proxy.

If we consider the *sources of moral authority of the proxy*, it becomes clear that they originate from what is known about the patient's wishes and the fact that the proxy was *chosen* by the patient. The first sort of moral authority is *substantive* or specific knowledge of the patient's wishes. The second is *procedural*. Here, being chosen as the designated surrogate invests the proxy with discretionary authority. Both sources of the proxy's moral authority stem from the patient's own expression of self-determination.[32]

So let us return to the case of the proxy who was told "to do everything, no matter what." In this case, we believe that the proxy would be entitled to exercise both her substantive and procedural moral authority in making a judgment. If the burdens were overwhelming and there was in reality, nothing or very little that could be achieved, the proxy would seem to be making a reasonable choice to forgo additional therapy. If it were more a judgment call about the efficacy of the proposed treatment, the proxy could reasonably opt for a time trial of therapy to see if any improvement might be achieved.

The point is not to tell you how to decide in cases such as these involving proxy decision makers. Instead, it is to suggest a way to recognize and respond to ethical tensions that may emerge when dealing with a proxy so as to optimize patient care and assist the proxy with the burdens associated with surrogate decision making. When interpreting these issues, it may be helpful to seek out the counsel of your hospital ethics committee. (See Chapter 9 for more details on the role of ethics committees.)

Withdrawals of Care

The decision to withdraw life-sustaining therapy, especially ventilatory support, is one of the most difficult choices a surrogate can make. It is difficult because surrogates and clinicians may feel that they are not withdrawing life-sustaining care but actually causing death.

As we discussed in Chapter 3, withdrawal of life-sustaining therapy is distinct from physician-assisted suicide. There is a clear legal and clinical consensus on this issue.[37,38] Central to this distinction is that there is a fundamental *causal* distinction between removing an impediment to death and engaging in an action which is both necessary and sufficient to cause death.

This will become clearer if we entertain a thought experiment. Consider two patients who require mechanical ventilation and are both sedated. The first patient has adult respiratory distress syndrome (ARDS). The second patient required general anesthesia for abdominal surgery. Sedation wears off on both patients and both are extubated. The patient with ARDS will die because he is ventilator dependent. The post-operative patient survives and breathes on his own. The difference in outcome is critical as we consider the moral significance of extubation as it relates to causing death.

Because the outcomes were different, it is clear that the act of extubation was *necessary but not sufficient* to cause death. Indeed it was the underlying disease process of ARDS that caused the first patient to die. The ventilator was an impediment to death, not its cause. As the philosopher Daniel Callahan has elegantly noted, ". . . only dying people will die when life support is removed, not those of us who are healthy." [39]

Here the removal of a ventilator only leads to the death of the patient who requires ventilatory support. Unlike assisted suicide, which does not hinge on an underlying illness to cause death, the removal of the ventilator leads to death only when there is an underlying disease process.[40]

Too often, the distinction between assisted suicide and withdrawals are not understood in the clinical context. This can cause a number of problematic situations. For example, an ambivalent attending physician who has not sorted these issues out for himself may delegate the task of extubation to you or a respiratory therapist. It is important that you ask for adequate emotional or clinical support in these circumstances. If your attending seems to be evasive, you should seek out the chief resident or another attending for assistance.

A second scenario is when a designated surrogate wants to withdraw care but does not want to remove the ventilator. For example, a decision is made to withdraw some elements of care, say dialysis and antibiotics, but to continue mechanical ventilation. When this happens death is prolonged and the patient dies of progressive uremia or sepsis while ventilatory support is maintained. An inevitable death, one that is expected and perhaps even hoped for by loving family, is delayed because no one was comfortable disconnecting a ventilator, even though other life-sustaining measures were withdrawn.

This occurs because the family or the clinician views the withdrawal of the ventilator differently because death will be more immediate with extubation than the withdrawal of dialysis. They reason, in my view erroneously, that since death is more immediate, extubation has caused the death and that the physician who ordered the cessation of ventilatory support is responsible.

A decision to remove a ventilator, or to discontinue chronic dialysis, is a morally weighty action that should be addressed with seriousness and studied attention. Nonetheless, it is important to avoid mistaking the gravity of the decision with its impermissibility.

Too often, our unresolved ambivalence about withdrawals of care are never articulated and brought to the surface. Hence, anytime a withdrawal of care is considered it is an appropriate time to address overall goals of care. If we do not engage in this more comprehensive assessment, we run the risk of providing inconsistent care that may prolong patient distress and the dying process contrary to patient or family preferences.

Hospice or Palliative Care Referral

We would hope that goals of care would have been discussed by the time a decision has been made to seek out palliative care or a hospice referral. Engaging in goal setting at this point in the course of illness, may be "too little, too late." Nonetheless, a decision to opt for hospice or palliative care is a good time to review overall goals of care and outline strategies to optimize patient and family well-being.

The first question that needs to be addressed is: what exactly do we mean by palliative or hospice care? In Chapter 1, we considered the history of the palliative care movement and current elements of care. Your challenge is how to translate these expectations to individual patients and their families. Each will understand palliative care differently.

Palliative care can also be context driven. In some places it is called supportive care; in others comfort care. Each practice pattern reflects local cultural dimensions as well as national guidelines.[41]

Although we envision palliative care as a comprehensive care strategy that seeks to relieve the patient's pain and symptom burden and attend to the broader psychosocial needs of patient and family, in some settings a designation of palliative or comfort care merely means that the level of current care will not be escalated. For example, a patient who is becoming hemodynamically unstable will *not* be transferred to the intensive care unit.

Some surrogates will be in favor of palliative care, but not hospice, because "that is where you go to die." For all these reasons, when caring for patients who are opting for palliation and/or hospice, it is important to be clear about definitions and expectations. Most importantly, it is necessary to dispel misconceptions about palliation and hospice, which may undermine decisions to pursue these important care options.

So how should we conceptualize comfort, supportive, or palliative care in the hospital setting? There are two essential elements. The first is the *refusal* of unwanted interventions like CPR, unit referral, or artificial nutrition and hydration. The second acknowledges the clinician's *affirmative obligations* to patients and families. This respects the refusal of curative care while it actively pursues pain and symptom management, psychosocial and spiritual support.

Some view the pursuit of palliation as the abandonment of any hope of cure. While palliation is generally provided to patients who are dying and have eluded cure, palliative care can also be a element of therapy for patients who are receiving active care. A patient with a treatable illness with associated comorbidity *should* be palliated even as a cure is pursued.

These *mosaic approaches* to palliative care seek to blend the most appropriate elements of care and cure. If we were to return to the figure on page 83, we see that palliative and curative interventions coexist throughout the trajectory of an illness. What changes is the *balance* of caring and curing.[42] This is important to stress to patients and families who may falsely believe that cure is being abandoned once palliation is broached.

There are a number of ways that palliative care is provided in the acute-care setting.[43] Although we hope that these skills will eventually be a basic competency of all clinicians, specialty units and services do exist in many hospitals to provide this care.

In some hospitals there are dedicated palliative care units where staff are trained to focus on palliative versus curative interventions. These especially designed units resemble in-patient hospices, both conceptually and environmentally and can be thought of as a safe haven against the technological imperative epitomized by the Intensive Care Unit. When advancing this idea, we called these in-patient palliative care units *alternative* care units to suggest that they could be a viable option for those who decided *not* to pursue intensive care at the end of life.[44]

When palliative care physicians are involved with care, it is important to determine who will be the attending physician.

Will it be the patient's oncologist who shepherded the patient through chemotherapy, the cardiologist who attended to the management of mitral valve replacement for rheumatic heart disease, or the palliative care physician? Although the palliative care physician may have more skill in the management of the symptomatology of refractory disease, it is generally disruptive to transfer care so late in the course of illness. The oncologist or cardiologist has been there through the patient's course and the force of that doctor–patient relationship should not be discounted or discontinued. Sharing responsibilities with a palliative care physician who can assist with consultation is a preferred approach.

Hospice Care

Some patients, able to be discharged from the hospital or who refuse to be hospitalized, will opt for hospice referral. The provision of hospice care is another dimension of palliation that is often misunderstood. We reviewed the historical and philosophical origins of the modern hospice movement in Chapter 2. Here, we will consider some of the practical issues that may help your patients receive hospice care.

There has been a Federal Medicare Hospice Benefit since 1983.[45] This is a comprehensive benefit that includes physician services and nursing care and assumes the costs of drugs and medical devices. Most hospice care is provided in the home but the benefit does cover the cost of inpatient and respite hospice care. Patients and families also receive counseling, social work assistance, and pastoral care, should they request it. Bereavement services are also available for survivors. When most recently surveyed, there were 3,200 hospice programs nationwide with nearly 900,000 patients enrolled each year.[46]

Patients can transfer out of traditional Medicare and receive the hospice benefit instead. Patients are eligible for enrollment if their physician attests that they are terminally-ill with a life expectancy of six months or less. Patients who exceed this expected life expectancy can have their enrollment renewed.[47]

Fraud and abuse investigations by the Inspector General of the Department of Health and Human Services about length of stay in hospice during the late 1990s have led physicians to be tentative with their prognostication and wait until late in the course of an illness to make a hospice referral. This is among the factors that have led to shorter hospice stays before and after the passage of the Balanced Budget Act of 1997.[48] Unfortunately, this has led to a high prevalence of patients with a short length of stay. In 2000, the mean length of hospice care was 46.9 days, and the median length of care was just 15.6 days with 63 percent of patients receiving care for less than 30 days.[49] In a separate study, 36 percent of patients referred to hospice from non-nursing home settings had an average length of less than eight days.[50] This is clearly too short a period to engage in comprehensive palliative care.[51]

This short length of stay also places a tremendous financial strain on hospice programs themselves because their funding is predicated upon patient enrollment for a six month period. Medicare pays hospice programs a per diem rate, a fixed amount of money per day of service provided. It is expected that costs of care will be less when the patient is first referred to hospice and then rise as the patient's illness progresses and the need for services increases. This economic model assumes that early periods of lower cost will help offset the higher costs of care nearer to the time of death.[52]

But because the length of stay in hospice is shifted towards the very end of life, hospice programs are unable to cost shift between periods of less and more cost. This entitlement structure asks hospice programs to choose between meeting their patients' needs and ensuring the financial viability of their programs.[53] This places an untenable burden on these programs and forces them to curtail services and engage in robust fundraising.[54]

When deciding about whether to refer a patient to a hospice, it is also important to consider whether the program is a not-for-profit or for-profit entity. Recent questions have arisen about the quality of care provided by some for-profit hospice companies, which are viewed by Wall Street as a growth industry, given national demographics and the aging of our population.[46]

References

1 Elpern EH, Yellen SB, and Burton LA. A Preliminary Investigation of Opinions and Behaviors Regarding Advance Directives for Medical Care. *American Journal of Critical Care* 2(2)(1993):161–167.

2 Romero LJ, Lindeman RD, Koenler KM, et al. Influence of Ethnicity on Advance Directives and End-of-life Decisions. *Journal of the American Medical Association*, 277(4)(1997):298–299.

3 Silveira MJ, DiPiero A, Gerrity MS, et al. Patient's Knowledge of Options at the End of Life. *Journal of the American Medical Association*, 284(19)(2000):2483–2488.

4 Cohen CB and Cohen PJ. Do-not-resuscitate Orders in the Operating Room. *New England Journal of Medicine* 325(26)(1991):1879–1882.

5 Statement of the American College of Surgeons on Advance Directives by Patients. 'Do Not Resuscitate' in the OR. *ACS Bulletin* (September 1994): 29.

6 Cotler MP. The 'Do-not-resuscitate' Order; Clinical and Ethical Rationale and Implications. *Medicine and Law* 19(3)(2000):623–33.

7 Murphy DJ, Burrows D, Santilli S, et al. The Influence of the Proba-bility of Survival on Patients' Preferences Regarding Cardiopulmonary Resuscitation. *New England Journal of Medicine* 330(8)(1994):545–9.

8 Crawley L, Payne R, Bolden J, et al. Initiative to Improve Palliative and End-of-Life Care in the African American Community. Palliative and End-of-life Care in the African American Community. *Journal of the American Medical Association* 284(19)(2000):2518–2521.

9 Lear MW. *Heartsounds.* New York: Random House, 1988.

10 Shepardson LB, Gordon HS, Ibrahim SA, et al. Racial Variation in the Use of Do-not-resuscitate Orders. *Journal of General Internal Medicine* 14(1)(1999):15–20.

11 Waters CM. Understanding and Supporting African Americans' Per-spectives of End-of-life Care Planning and Decision Making. *Qualita-tive Health Research* 11(3)(2001):385–398.

12 Fins JJ. Vowing to Care. *Journal of Pain and Symptom Management* 23(1)(2002):54–57.

13 Abraham LK. Life-Sustaining Technology. In *Mama Might be Better off Dead.* Chicago: The University of Chicago Press, 1993, 213–231.

14 Williams JF, Zimmerman JE, Wagner DP, et al. African-American and White Patients Admitted to the Intensive Care Unit: Is There a Differ-ence in Therapy and Outcome? *Critical Care Medicine* 23(4)(1995): 626–636.

15 Berger JT. Ethical Challenges of Partial Do-Not-Resuscitate (DNR) Orders. *Archives of Internal Medicine* 163(19)(2003):2270–2275.

16 Dumot JA, Burval DJ, Sprung J, et al. Outcome of Adult Cardiopul-monary Resuscitations at a Tertiary Referral Center Including Results of "Limited" Resuscitations. *Archives of Internal Medicine* 161(14) (2001):1751–1758.

17 Wolf SM. Patient Self-Determination Act. Honoring Broader Direc-tives. *Hastings Center Report* 21(5)(1991):S8–9.

18 Miles SH, Koepp R, Weber EP. Advance End-of-life Treatment Plan-ning: A Research Review. *Archives of Internal Medicine* 156(10)(1996):1062-1068.

19 Hayward RS, Steinberg EP, Ford DE, et al. Preventive Care Guidelines: 1991. American College of Physicians. Canadian Task Force on the Periodic Health Examination. United States Preventive Services Task Force. *Annals of Internal Medicine* 114(9)(1991):758–783.

20 Wolf SM, Barondess JA, Boyle P, et al. Special Report: Sources of Con-cern About the Patient Self-Determination Act. *New England Journal of Medicine* 325(23):1666–1671.

21 Emanuel LL. Advance Directives: Do they Work? *Journal of the American College of Cardiology* 25(1)(1995):35–38.

22 Ott BB. Advance Directives: The Emerging Body of Research. *American Journal of Critical Care* 8(1)(1999):514–519.

23 Teno JM, Stevens M, Spernak S, et al. Role of Written Advance Directives in Decision Making: Insights from Qualitative and Quantitative Data. *Journal of General Internal Medicine* 13(7)(1998):439–446.

24 Teno JM, Licks S, Lynn J, et al. Do Advance Directives Provide Instructions That Direct Care? *Journal of the American Geriatric Society* 45(4)(1997):508–512.

25 Campbell ML. Interpretation of an Ambiguous Advance Directive. *Dimensions of Critical Care Nursing* 14(5)(1995):226–232.

26 Brett AS. Limitations of Listing Specific Medical Interventions in Advance Directives. *Journal of the American Medical Association* 266(6)(1991):825–828.

27 Danis M, Southerland LI, Garrett JM, et al. A Prospective Study of Advance Directives for Life-Sustaining Care. *New England Journal of Medicine* 324(13)(1991):882–888.

28 Maltby BS and Fins JJ. Informing the Patient-proxy Covenant: An Educational Approach for Advance Care Planning. *Innovations in End-of-Life Care* 5(2)(2003). www.edc.org/lastacts. Reprinted as Maltby BS, Fins JJ. Informing the Patient-proxy Covenant: An Educational Approach for Advance Care Planning. *Journal of Palliative Medicine* 7(2)(2004):351–55.

29 Fins JJ and Maltby BS. *Fidelity, Wisdom, and Love: Patients and Proxies in Partnership, Interactive Workbook and Educational Video.* New York: Fan Fox and Leslie R. Samuels Foundation, 2003.

30 Fins JJ, Maltby BS, Friedmann E, et al. Contracts, Covenants and Advance Care Planning: An Empirical Study of the Moral Obligations of Patient and Proxy. *Journal of Pain and Symptom Management* 29(1)(2005):55–68.

31 Fins JJ. The Patient Self-Determination Act and Patient-Physician Collaboration in New York State. *New York State Journal of Medicine* 92(11)(1992):489–493.

32 Fins JJ. From Contract to Covenant in Advance Care Planning. *Journal of Law, Medicine & Ethics* 27(1)(1999):46–51.

33 Emanuel L. PSDA in the Clinic. *Hastings Center Report* 21(5)(1991):S6–7.

34 The New York State Public Health Law, Article 29-C. Health Care Proxy Law 2982.2.

35 Brock DW. Trumping Advance Directives. *Hastings Center Report* 21(5)(1991):S5–6.

36 Singer P, Martin DK, Lavery JU, et al. Reconceptualizing Advance Care Planning from the Patient's Perspective. *Archives of Internal Medicine* 158(8)(1997):879–884.

37 Kamissar Y. In Defense of the Distinction between Terminating Life Support and Actively Intervening to Promote or Bring about Death. *BioLaw* 2(7&8)(1996):S145–S149.

38 Miller FG, Fins JJ, and Snyder L. Assisted Suicide and Refusal of Treatment: Valid Distinction? *Annals of Internal Medicine* 132(6)(2000): 470–475.

39 Callahan D. Physician-Assisted Suicide: Opening the Poor to Moral Mischief. *Newsday*. April 11, 1996.

40 Fins JJ. Principles in Palliative Care: An Overview. *Journal of Respiratory Care* 45(11)(2000):1320–1330.

41 Fins JJ, Peres JR, Schumacher JD, and Meier C. *On the Road from Theory to Practice: A Resource Guide to Promising Practices in Palliative Care Near the End of Life*. Washington, DC: Last Acts National Program Office, Robert Wood Johnson Foundation, 2003.

42 Numbers RL and Amundsen DW. *Caring and Curing*. New York: Macmillan, 1986.

43 Pan CX, Morrison RS, Meier DE, et al. How Prevalent are Hospital-based Palliative Care Programs? Status Report and Future Directions. *Journal of Palliative Medicine* 4(3)(2001):315–324.

44 Miller FG and Fins JJ. A Proposal to Restructure Hospital Care for Dying Patients. *New England Journal of Medicine* 334(26)(1996): 1740–1742.

45 Hoyer T. A History of the Medicare Hospice Benefit. *The Hospice Journal* 13(1-2)(1998):61–69.

46 Ward S. Troubling Odyssey. Questions Arise about Hospice Company's Patient Care, Level of Medicare Payments. *Barron's* April 12, 2004: 20–22.

47 National Hospice Organization. *Hospice Fact Sheet*. Arlington, VA: National Hospice Organization, Summer 1998.

48 Murkofsky RL, Phillips RS, McCarthy EP, et al. Length of Stay in Home Care Before and After the 1997 Balanced Budget Act. *Journal of the American Medical Association* 289(21)(2003):2841–2848.

49 Haupt BJ. "Characteristics of Hospice Care Discharges and Their Length of Service: United States, 2000. *Vital Health Stat* 13 (154) (2003):1–36.

50 Miller SC, Weitzen S, and Kinzbrunner B. Factors Associated with the High Prevalence of Short Hospice Stays. *Journal of Palliative Medicine* 6(5)(2003):725–736.

51 Miller SC, Kinzbrunner B, Pettit P, et al. How Does the Timing of Hospice Referral Influence Hospice Care in the Last Days of Life? *Journal of the American Geriatric Society* 51(6)(2003):798–806.

52 Attorney General Dennis C. Vacco's Commission on Quality Care at the End of Life. *Final Report*. Albany, NY: Office of the Attorney General of New York State. July, 1998.

53 Byock IR. A Consensus Statement by Radiation Oncologists Regarding Radiotherapy for Bone Metastases. *American Journal of Hospice and Palliative Care* 9(5)(1992)6–7.

54 Fins JJ. The Limitations of Hospice. *The Cortland Forum* 6(3)(1993):46.

c h a p t e r   e i g h t

Goals of Care: Medical Developments

Introduction

The premise of this chapter is that we need to overcome the routinization of care and our reflexive response to clinical developments. It is appropriate that the patient who develops respiratory distress receives ventilatory support but a decision to escalate care is inappropriate if we fail to ask whether the introduction of life-sustaining therapy is consistent with the patient's preferences and goals. In this chapter, we will consider clinical developments that should prompt a reconsideration of the goals of care and a more critical assessment of the therapeutic response to life-threatening developments.

Figure 8-1   Medical Developments

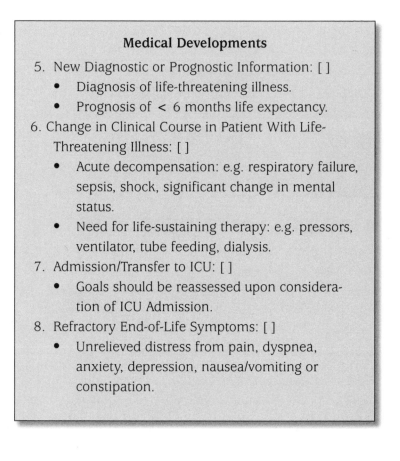

Medical Developments

5. New Diagnostic or Prognostic Information: [ ]
   - Diagnosis of life-threatening illness.
   - Prognosis of < 6 months life expectancy.
6. Change in Clinical Course in Patient With Life-Threatening Illness: [ ]
   - Acute decompensation: e.g. respiratory failure, sepsis, shock, significant change in mental status.
   - Need for life-sustaining therapy: e.g. pressors, ventilator, tube feeding, dialysis.
7. Admission/Transfer to ICU: [ ]
   - Goals should be reassessed upon consideration of ICU Admission.
8. Refractory End-of-Life Symptoms: [ ]
   - Unrelieved distress from pain, dyspnea, anxiety, depression, nausea/vomiting or constipation.

A Life-Threatening Illness

New diagnostic or prognostic information should cause you to reconsider the goals of care. This is routine in the curative paradigm but often overlooked when patients are near the end of life. In these cases we often respond tactically to new information. An elderly patient is diagnosed with non-Hodgkins lymphoma after developing an ileus which shows a near total bowel obstruction. Although the chances of cure exist with chemotherapy—and should be pursued—the possibility that there will be a fatal outcome should prompt a reconsideration of the goals of care.

At this juncture it is quite reasonable to pursue *both* curative and palliative goals. At the time of diagnosis, it is too early to know how the patient will fare and the course the illness will take. Neither the physician nor the patient knows how responsive the tumor will be to chemotherapy. Statistics will give a general sense of response rate for all patients with this disease, but can not tell us how a particular patient will fare.

This uncertainty can lead to distortions in judgment that can lead to therapeutic hype or inappropriate resignation. An overly optimistic oncologist might say to a patient that, "only 5 percent of patients with this illness will survive, but if you're one of those 5 percent, it's 100 percent for you." Clearly, this is disingenuous and misrepresents the patient's odds for a good outcome. The pessimistic clinician might leap prematurely to a palliative course because of unfavorable odds. Despite our efforts to advance palliation, it would be inappropriate to withhold potentially curative therapy upon diagnosis, even if cure is elusive. While the patient may refuse to pursue this course, it is paternalistic for the physician to make a judgment to withhold therapy unilaterally.

When the prognosis is dire, it seems best to embrace dual goals of care at the beginning—to seek cure *and* to minimize the burdens associated with such care. This will not only avoid unrealistic expectations and potential futility disputes but help the patient maximize the benefits of therapy while limiting therapy-related toxicity.

The patient should be helped to hope for the best but be prepared for the worst. They should receive aggressive treatments that will hopefully result in cure while you also have a frank discussion about the more likely outcome. Ideally, the possibility of an adverse outcome should be introduced early in the course of care so the patient will have time to express preferences before losing the opportunity to do so. This process could be initiated with a conversation about advance care planning.

Unfortunately, many clinicians are hesitant to bring up adverse outcomes. They worry that it sends the wrong message. Or they feel that it would be cruel to further burden the patient with these concerns; that it is too much to handle during an early visit. While there is some merit to that argument, too often the conversation is delayed and does not occur until after the patient has lost capacity. This robs the patient of an opportunity to articulate preferences and leaves the surrogate with the burden of having to elect a course of care without discussion with the patient about preferences.

Another occasion for dialogue is when a treatment failure turns a hopeful diagnosis into one with an unfavorable outcome. For example, care is initiated for a treatable cancer. The patient is unresponsive to chemotherapy and another more toxic and experimental agent is tried. This is a bad prognostic sign and an occasion to ask whether curative goals of care are still attainable. While it is still reasonable to seek a cure and try a new course of therapy, this should be tempered by a growing realization that it may be necessary to shift the focus of care.

Each of these occasions should trigger a consideration or reconsideration of the goals of care. Early conversation will provide the patient with time to make plans. If treatment does not succeed, it will provide you with deeper insights into a patient who will increasingly depend upon you for care.

Prognosis

In order to consider treatment options and goals of care, we must have a sense of what to expect from the disease or condition, and how much time there will be before the patient dies. According to the Oxford English Dictionary, a prognosis is, "A forecast of the probable course and termination of a case of disease" or "the action or art of making such a forecast."[1]

Prognosis is probabilistic and exceedingly difficult. Because of its uncertainty, explicit mention of prognosis is often left out of discussions about treatment decisions although such information is needed to satisfy the doctrine of informed consent.[2]

Studies have shown that prognostication is far from an exact science. In many cases the physician's best guess has been shown to be no more accurate than a coin toss.[3] In the SUPPORT study of critically ill patients, for example, physicians were unable to predict which cohort of patients would be alive after six months.[4] Despite an abundance of physical evidence, laboratory and radiographic data, a literature of survival rates and disease processes, plus professional experience and intuition, it is difficult to accurately predict what will happen and when death will occur. Not surprisingly, many physicians avoid doing so. They do not want to take the risk of being wrong.

Studies of prognostic accuracy in cancer patients have generally found that physicians were "accurate" (accurate being liberally defined as within 33 percent of observed survival) 10–30 percent of the time. Interestingly, the majority of these physicians overestimated survival time.[3] Similar studies of intensive care unit physicians found that they tended to be more pessimistic in their predictions, but they, too, were way off base more often than not.[3] It is no wonder then, that so many physicians avoid communicating a prognosis to patients and families, even though they are frequently asked to do so.[5]

Because patients with a prognosis of six months or less are eligible for hospice enrollment, that milestone is an important occasion to reconsider goals of care, acknowledging the difficulty of even getting this crude prognosis correct.

The National Hospice Organization has grappled with the same problem because of the hospice eligibility question and developed a series of guidelines for several diseases that establish a prognosis of 6 months or less. For example, a patient with pulmonary disease, who experiences disabling dyspnea, FEV1 < 30%, frequent emergencies, cor pulmonale, hypoxemia on O2, hypercapnea, resting tachycardia, or unintended weight loss, is deemed to have a prognosis of < 6 months.[6] Despite their fallibility, guidelines such as this may be useful in establishing a prognosis and engage in structured goal setting.

A lack of accurate predictors of outcome is only part of the challenge. Physician bias is another. Physicians bring their own hopes and aspirations for their patients to prognostication and this can distort their objectivity.[7] In addition, patients and physicians can collude in "false optimism" about an anticipated "recovery plot" that does not cohere with the objective reality of their illness.[8]

Because prognosis is uncertain and open to bias and false hope, frank conversation about end-of-life care seldom takes place until the very end of the patient's life. (As we have discussed, over 80 percent of patients are made DNR by a surrogate because discourse with the patient has been delayed.) By using a trigger of six months to prompt dialogue we do not mean to suggest that conversations should not occur sooner. We are simply hoping that they will have occurred by that time.

In some disease trajectories, a first conversation at six months would be too late. For example in progressive Alzheimer's disease, six months before death a patient will be unable to express her preferences and may have already experienced care which was disproportionate given constricted life expectancy and cognitive impairment.[9]

Having considered all this, what should be your response to the patient or family who asks about prognosis: "How much time is left?" While prognostication becomes more predictable as death becomes imminent, it is best to be frank and acknowledge the difficulties with prediction while reaffirming your commitment to the patient's well-being. After asking about patient or family expectations, you should consult the literature about outcomes and use this to inform your comments. When conveying a prognosis you should be sensitive to patient and family expectations.

For example, if a family is more optimistic than clinically warranted, you might help them accept a more ominous prognosis by allowing them to come to it over time. A prognosis delivered prematurely may cause distress or even engender conflict. It is better to help prepare patient and family for this information.

Consider the patient on a ventilator with a post-obstructive pneumonia and advanced lung cancer. The family asks how long the patient has to be on the ventilator. You sense that they hope to receive promising news. For this expectant family, you might suggest that the patient's "prognosis looks less good, the longer he or she stays on the ventilator." You might suggest that, "Let's see how he does over the weekend" and reconvene the conversation the following week.

Although you believe that the patient will not be extubatable in two days, you have given the family members the opportunity to come to this same realization on their own.[10]

Let time be an elixir that allows the family to appreciate what you already know about the patient's chances. Over the weekend, they will see that the patient is unable to be weaned. When the ventilator settings are increased they will better appreciate the patient's condition. By Monday, they will be in a better position to hear your prognosis and its implications.

Even when you can assert an evidence-based prognosis, you should still be cautious in your statements. They should be *tempered with humility*. Although you may believe that this acknowledgement betrays a lack of knowledge, families will appreciate your honesty and thoughtfulness.

Failure to be correct with a prognosis delivered with certainty is a harbinger of a futility dispute. If you were wrong once in predicting a dire outcome, the next time you lay out a futile scenario the patient or family may not trust you. (See Chapter 4 for more on futility.)

Conversely, if you are able to predict that death is coming, you can moderate expectations. This was something that Hippocrates noted in his *Prognosis*, "By realizing and announcing beforehand which patients were going to die, he [the physician] would absolve himself of any blame."[11]

Ultimately, a question such as "how much time is left?" is a deeper question that requires more than a forecast in weeks or months. The patient or family member who asks that question is communicating to you an anticipatory sense of loss or implicitly asking about the current goals of care. Their question should be perceived as a call for help and viewed as an opening to ask them about their expectations, unfinished business and unfulfilled hopes that may yet be completed and realized.

Acute Decompensation and the Use of Life-Sustaining Therapies

Acute decompensation in very ill patients is accompanied by considerable increases in morbidity and mortality. It can also herald new insights and fundamentally alter the patient's, family's, and staff's perception of the gravity of the situation. The patient may view the disease differently as the possibility of death becomes more real. Hopeful families may begin to realize that a cure may no longer be possible. And staff, too, may have their doubts.

Consider the patient with multiple myeloma admitted for chemotherapy who develops a fungal pneumonia, thus transforming a "routine" admission into one that places the patient's life in jeopardy. This life-threatening development will shift the *focus* of care, but will it change the *goals* of care? Had the patient and the family previously considered this development? Were they aware of this potential complication? Do they understand what this change in condition means and the new burdens of care that treatment of a fungal pneumonia entails?

The development of a fungal pneumonia is more than an infection, it is also an *inflection point in the patient's disease trajectory* that should prompt a discussion about the goals of care. As a disease progresses, each subsequent need for life-sustaining therapy requires a fresh evaluation of goals and meaning.

Consideration of ICU Transfer

We considered the culture of intensive care in Chapter 4. In this section, we will focus solely on decisions to transfer patients to the ICU. An ICU transfer should be seen, not simply as a change in venue, but an intervention in and of itself. After all, the patient is being moved to the ICU because of its potential to provide a bundle of therapies that are not available elsewhere in the hospital.

Nonetheless, we tend not to think of an ICU admission as an intervention that requires informed consent. Although we routinely obtain consent for procedures like a line placement or a blood transfusion, we often *assume* that consent is implied when it comes to a unit transfer.

Certainly, part of this could be explained by the urgency of many ICU admissions and the inability to have discussions until the patient is more stable. Seen in this light, this deferral of discussion is consistent with an *emergency presumption* that allows for the provision of life-saving interventions when the patient can not provide consent. As we noted in Chapter 2, this was articulated by the jurist Benjamin Cardozo in 1914 in the landmark *Schloendorff* decision. He asserted that informed consent is necessary from adult competent patients, "except in cases of emergency when the patient is unconscious and when it is necessary to operate before consent can be obtained."[12]

But, even in cases involving a stable patient, informed consent for ICU transfer is rarely obtained. Most likely, this stems from the perception of the team that ICU care is not a treatment choice but a necessity—a natural escalation of care. At these times, clinicians must pause to consider whether or not that treatment plan continues to be aligned with the patient's treatment goals.

This is especially important because much narrative information can be lost as patients move from a regular medical floor to the ICU and a new medical team. Both the family and the team will be burdened with starting from scratch. While being preoccupied with emergency management of a life-threatening complication, this new team will need to establish a rapport with the patient and the family and begin to develop a new therapeutic relationship. Initiating a new doctor–patient–family relationship is difficult under any circumstances but especially challenging given the stress of an ICU admission. For this reason, structured goal setting during this time can be particularly helpful.

Symptoms at the End of Life

Patients with terminal illness suffer chronically with many symptoms. One large multi-center study of cancer patients found that 51 percent experienced moderate to severe pain. Other common symptoms included weakness (51 percent), weight loss (39 percent), anorexia (30 percent), constipation (23 percent), nausea (21 percent), and dyspnea (19 percent).[13] This study did not include the symptoms of depression and anxiety, which are also common among the terminally ill.[14]

Our objective here is not to instruct you in the management of these problems—other texts can do that[15]—but rather to help you reconceptualize how we assess these symptoms in patients who are dying. In contrast to acute care medicine focused on cure, diagnosis dictates the treatment that follows.[16] In palliative care, loss of function dictates what care is needed.

When clinicians think in conventional diagnostic terms, a nuanced diagnostic distinction can be very important. For example, differentiating between legionella or pneumococcal pneumonia is a critical distinction in determining which antibiotic is chosen. In palliative medicine, diagnostic assessment differs. It is less important how your patient became incontinent or lost mobility than to recognize that function has been lost. Incontinence from a stroke, normal pressure hydrocephalus, or a spinal cord injury all have a common final pathway—the need for supportive services. While the diagnosis and etiology of the disability is not without importance, it is the functional loss or burden of illness that determines patient needs in palliative care. Here the focus is on the symptom and not its genesis, unless that knowledge will help to mitigate distress or restore function.

Symptom burden near the end of life should also prompt a consideration of what ethicists call *proportionality*, the proportion of benefits to burdens. If we consider benefits versus burdens as a fraction, Benefits/Burdens, is there a net benefit to the patient? Would that fraction be > 1, meaning that the benefits were greater than the burdens? Or would the symptom burden be so significant that the fraction is < 1? Although it may be difficult to quantify this relationship of benefits to burdens, conceptualizing them together as a proportion can help you and your patients make more informed choices. What is important is to not discount patient distress or inflate the likelihood of cure when you engage in analysis. Either action could lead to the pursuit of disproportionate care.

The Ethics of Opioid Use

In considering symptom burden we should also discuss their relief and the ethical dilemmas posed by the use of opioid analgesia. Although you have been instructed in preclinical courses in pharmacology and medical ethics to use opioids to treat pain, these educational gains in palliative care are often reversed in the clinical years.[17-19]

Unfortunately, what we preach is not always what we practice[20], and national studies demonstrate the continued under treatment of pain.[21,22] Although the relief of pain and suffering is accepted as a compelling ethical obligation, we continue to undertreat our patients. Although you will graduate from medical school with an ability to prescribe antibiotics, many students do not learn how to prescribe opioids for pain and symptom management[23] or they underestimate the patient's perception of pain and under treat.[24,25]

There are many reasons for this educational deficiency. They include unfounded fears that the use of these agents will cause addiction, regulatory impediments, and restrictive laws that impede access to needed medication.[26,27] If we consider the use of opioid analgesia at the end of life, we will find that many clinicians are reluctant to use sufficient dosages of these drugs because they fear their use may hasten death. If you want to be an advocate for your patient's pain relief you need to be able to articulate the arguments for better pain relief. This will help you urge your colleagues to engage in appropriate pain management and dispel your own reservations.

If we start with the law, the U.S. Supreme Court unequivocally affirmed the physician's obligation to relieve pain even if doing so may hasten an inevitable death. (See Chapter 3 for a discussion of judicial ruling on assisted suicide and palliative care.)[28] The *doctrine of double effect* was invoked in this legal justification.

Double effect is an important construct for you to know. It is an argument from moral theology first introduced by Saint Thomas Aquinas, which distinguishes primary intentions and secondary effects.[29] In the context of end-of-life care, it helps to distinguish interventions that relieve suffering that may hasten death from physician-assisted suicide or euthanasia when death is intended.[30] With respect to the use of a morphine drip hung to treat a patient's pain, the dose needed to treat a patient's pain may also—as a secondary, unintended, or double effect—suppress respiratory function and so hasten the patient's death. But unlike physician-assisted suicide where the intention is to end a life, the intention with a morphine drip is to treat pain and not cause death. In this case the dose is calibrated to the patient's level of pain and discomfort. This is philosophically distinguished in law and ethics from euthanasia in which a large enough dose of morphine able to cause death is given intentionally.

But as you will see on the wards, this philosophical *bright line distinction* does not always hold up in clinical practice. It is a bit more ambiguous. Most physicians have ordered a morphine drip for patients and carefully titrated the amount of medication to treat the patient's pain and then been informed that the patient had died. The physician may not have intended the patient's death but is nonetheless grateful and relieved that the patient's ordeal is over. Does this mean that the death was intended? Does it suggest that the physician used the doctrine of double effect as justification for an inappropriate action? Or was it invoked to promote the unequivocal good of pain relief?

Double effect can help allay the concern of physicians that they are both culpable and causal agents when a terminally-ill patient dies while receiving opioid analgesia. The use of double effect, though philosophically imperfect, has had great instrumental value in clinical practice and the law.[31] It helps the anxious practitioner use opioids more liberally in terminally-ill patients by highlighting the moral distinction between intended consequences and ones that were foreseeable but unintended.[32]

Unfortunately, the utility of double effect at the bedside and in the law, has fallen prey to an ideological battle over the ethical propriety of physician-assisted suicide. Advocates of legalization have sought to equate double effect with assisted suicide in order to legitimize assisted death.[33] These rhetorical efforts to deconstruct double effect have heightened physician reluctance to use opioids and undermined the security afforded by this philosophical formulation.[32]

References

1 *Oxford English Dictionary*, 2nd edition. New York: Oxford University Press, 1989.

2 Rich BA. Defining and Delineating a Duty to Prognosticate. *Theoretical Medicine* 22(3)(2001):177–192.

3 Christakis, NA. *Death Foretold: Prophecy and Prognosis in Medical Care.* Chicago: The University of Chicago Press, 2001.

4 The SUPPORT Principal Investigators. A Controlled Trial to Improve Care for Seriously Ill Hospitalized Patients. *Journal of the American Medical Association* 274(20)(1995): 1591–1598.

5 Christakis NA and Iwashyna TJ. Attitude and Self-reported Practice Regarding Prognostication in a National Sample of Internists. *Archives of Internal Medicine*, 158(21)(1998):2389–2395.

6 Stuart B, Alexander C, Arenella C, et al. *Medical Guidelines for Determining Prognosis in Selected Non-Cancer Disease*, ed. 2. Arlington, VA: National Hospice Organization, 1996.

7 Becker RB and Zimmerman JE. ICU Scoring Systems Allow Prediction of Patient Outcomes and Comparison of ICU Performance. *Critical Care Clinic* 12(3)(1996):503–514.

8 The AM, Hak T, Koeter G, et al. Collusion in Doctor-patient Communication about Imminent Death: An Ethnographic Study. *British Medical Journal* 321(7273)(2000):1376–1381.

9 Raik BL, Miller FG and Fins JJ. Screening and Cognitive Impairment: Ethics of Forgoing Mammography in Older Women. *Journal of the American Geriatrics Society* 52(3)(2004):440–444.

10 Fins JJ. A 38-year-old Man with a Secondary Leukemia who Needs Setting of Goals of Care. In Heffner JE and Byock I (Eds.) *Palliative and End-of-Life Pearls*. Philadelphia: Hanley and Belfus, 2002: 174–176.

11 Lloyd GER, Editor. *Hippocratic Writings*. Prognosis. New York:Penguin Books, 1983: 170.

12 *Schloendorff v Society of New York Hosp.*, 211 N.Y. 125 (1914).

13 Vaino A and Auvinen A. Prevalence of Symptoms Among Patients with Advanced Cancer: An International Collaborative Study. *Journal of Pain and Symptom Management* 12(1)(1996):3–10.

14 Breitbart W and Jacobsen PB. Psychiatric Symptom Management in Terminal Care. *Clinics in Geriatric Medicine* 12(2)(1996):329–347.

15 Doyle D, Hanks GWC, and MacDonald N. *Oxford Textbook of Palliative Medicine*, 2nd edition. New York: Oxford University Press, 1998.

16 Fins JJ. An Acute Care Response to Chronic Care: The American Perspective. *Journal of Czech Physicians* 132(7)(1993):197–199.

17 Barnard D, Quill T, Hafferty FW, et al. Preparing the Ground: Contributions of the Preclinical Years to Medical Education for Care Near the End of Life. *Academic Medicine* 74(5)(1999):499–505.

18 Block S and Billings A. Nurturing Humanism Through Teaching Palliative Care. *Academic Medicine* 73(7)(1998):763–765.

19 Fins JJ, Gentilesco BJ, Carver A, et al. Reflective Practice and Palliative Care Education: A Clerkship Responds to the Informal and Hidden Curriculum. *Academic Medicine* 78(3)(2003):307–312.

20 Foley KM. Pain Relief into Practice: Rhetoric without Reform. *Journal of Clinical Oncology* 13(9)(1995):2149–2151.

21 Cherny NI and Catane R. Professional Negligence in the Management of Cancer Pain: A Case for Urgent Reforms. *Cancer* 76(11)(1995): 2181–2185.

22 Committee on Care at the End of Life, Field MJ and Cassel CK, editors. *Approaching Death: Improving Care at the End of Life.* Washington, DC. Institute of Medicine–National Academy Press, 1997.

23 Fins JJ and Nilson EG. An Approach to Educating Residents about Palliative Care and Clinical Ethics. *Academic Medicine* 75(6)(2000): 662–665.

24 Drayer RA, Henderson J and Reidenberg M. Barriers to Better Pain Control in Hospitalized Patients. *Journal of Pain and Symptom Management* 17(6)(1999): 434–440.

25 Nekolaichuk CL, Bruera E, Spachynski K, et al. A Comparison of Patient and Proxy Symptom Assessments in Advanced Cancer Patients. *Palliative Medicine* 13(4)(1999): 311–323.

26 Hill CS Jr. The Barriers to Adequate Pain Management with Opioid Analgesics. *Seminars in Oncology* 20(2 suppl 1)(1993):1–5.

27 Reidenberg MM. Barriers to Controlling Pain in Patients with Cancer. *Lancet* 347(9011)(1996):1278.

28 Burt RA. The Supreme Court Speaks—Not Assisted Suicide but a Constitutional Right to Palliative Care. *New England Journal of Medicine* 337(17)(1997): 1234–1236.

29 Beauchamp TL and Childress JF. *Principles of Biomedical Ethics*, 4th ed. New York: Oxford University Press, 1994. pp. 206–211.

30 Part of this section is drawn from: Fins JJ. What Medicine and the Law Should do for the Physician-Assisted Suicide Debate. *CCAR Journal* 44(2)(1997):46–53

31 Miller FG, Fins JJ, and Snyder L. Assisted Suicide and Refusal of Treatment: Valid Distinction? *Annals of Internal Medicine* 132(6) (2000):470–475.

32 Fins JJ. Principles in Palliative Care: An Overview. *Journal of Respiratory Care* 45(11)(2000):1320–1330.

33 Quill TE. Principle of Double Effect and End-of-Life Management: Additional Myths and a Limited Role. *Journal of Palliative Medicine* 1(4)(1998):333–336.

chapter nine

Goal-Setting: Gathering Information

Introduction

Although it is critical to recognize the triggers that should initiate the process of goal setting, that recognition is but the first step to meeting the needs of patients and families. In this chapter, we will consider what information you will need to collect to be able to formulate goals of care. The information we will ask you to collect is both clinical and narrative, reflecting both medical circumstances and the broader psychosocial needs of patient and family.

Sources of Information

This information is sometimes easy to access from simply reading the chart.[1] More likely, though, you will need to seek out other sources of data because the medical record can be found lacking. Much of the information you will need will come from additional conversations with patients and their families and from nurses, social workers, chaplains, physical therapists, and other members of the interdisciplinary team caring for your patient.

It is important to remember that clinicians write the medical record from their perspective.[2] Given its authorship, the medical record may not accurately reflect the experiences of patients and families and the quality of care.[3] The disconnect between what we record in the medical record and what may be truly happening is captured in the pithy comment of Dr. Eugene Stead who observed on rounds, "I have nothing to add. Patient says she is feeling better and her chart seems to agree with this."[4] The admonition is clear. Dr. Stead warns us not to mistake clinical reality with our description of it in the medical record.[5] With this in mind, let us turn to the GCAT.

CLINICAL ASSESSMENT

TO BE COMPLETED BY PRIMARY CARE-GIVER
(HOUSE OFFICER, NURSE PRACTITIONER,
OR ATTENDING PHYSICIAN)

Name: _____ Age: _____

Hospital # _____

Today's Date: _____ Date of Admission: _____

Floor: _____ Service: _____

Attending: _____

Diagnosis: _____

Figure 9.1

Demographics and Local Culture

We generally do not pay much attention to basic demographic information. It gets a cursory glance. But even the simplest data can be valuable. Consider the elderly patient who comes into the hospital from home and is now unconscious and is on the brink of a unit transfer. She lives alone, is believed to have no family and her past medical history is unknown. A decision about care needs to be made. You look at her demographic information for a clue and notice that she has an old medical record number. You call for her chart and find the name of her internist who knows her well and her wishes regarding life-sustaining therapy.

Because a patient's length of stay can have a bearing on futility disputes (see Chapter 4), it is important to note when the patient was admitted and how long the hospitalization has been. And the longer the patient has been hospitalized, the greater the likelihood that care has become fragmented. Discontinuity of care can separate patients from their primary care physicians as the patient moves from one service to another.[6] With each transfer there is a loss of vital information about the patient and her preferences and often a fracturing of relationships with a favored nurse or house officer.

In some cases, it might even be difficult to *find* the older volumes of the patient's chart if she has been in the hospital for months. But these are the charts that you must read to understand the patient's history and to avoid missing details about their care that will be critical to helping with the formulation of meaningful goals.

Knowledge of the patient's floor and service may also be helpful in placing the patient's care into your institution's cultural context. Each floor and service has its own objectives and norms. While specialized care settings, like oncology units, ICUs, or hospice, help to cluster expertise and generally promote patient welfare, we need to remind ourselves that our view of what constitutes "appropriate care" is determined, in part, by the ethical norms of where it is given and received and who is providing it.[6]

Paradoxically, even laudatory institutional norms can disempower patients and families by dictating the discourse, or engineering expectations,[7] thereby altering expectations through the "bureaucratization of prognosis."[8] You need only to consider a patient with end-stage ischemic cardiomyopathy receiving aggressive care on the cardiothoracic care unit to appreciate this point. That unit is ideally suited to provide post-operative care but is itself a barrier to the provision of palliative care.

A major determinant of how care will proceed will be determined by the specialty, practice style, and personality of the attending physician. So it is critical for you to know with whom you will be working. Some attendings are philic to palliative care and incorporate this ethos into their practice. Others are death-phobic and avoid the mere mention of death and dying at all costs.

Working as an ethics consultant, I have seen this range of views. Disputes over end-of-life decisions that are *prevented* by some practitioners are *caused* by others. As a medical student or resident you need to know with whom you are working. Resident stress levels can escalate when they have to assume responsibility for end-of-life care when the attending has either abdicated this responsibility or is reluctant to let go.[9,10]

You should try to emulate attendings who are skilled in end-of-life care and help the patients of those who are not. In either case, you need to assess what sort of team you are on.

The Power of Diagnosis

There are a few things doctors can do that are more profound and life shaping than the act of diagnosis. With your knowledge of disease and illness, presentation and symptoms, you are able to confer a name upon what the patient has experienced and what you have observed. This is a power that needs to be wielded with great care because your pronouncements are easily open to misconstrual.

Making a diagnosis orders the world and creates expectations. A diagnosis is a unifying concept that brings clarity to a cluster of mysterious symptoms that may seem unrelated to each other in the mind of the patient. Using your diagnostic skills, you transform seemingly unrelated complaints into a single diagnosis. Symptoms like fatigue, edema, and muscle aches are understood as anemia and renal failure and lytic lesions. These findings coalesce into a diagnosis of multiple myeloma.

Although a diagnosis paves the way for a therapeutic intervention, it also confers meaning. The patient can no longer write off his fatigue from working too hard or edema from being on his feet too long. Muscle aches aren't because he is out of shape. Your diagnosis has transformed his world into the world of the sick.[11]

You know that a diagnosis of Congestive Heart Failure with a class IV Killip classification is a far more ominous diagnosis than a Dukes A Colon Cancer, though most lay persons would prefer to have "heart disease" over a diagnosis of cancer. So with the physician's prerogative of diagnosis comes the responsibility to educate, inform, and contextualize diagnostic information.

Osler once cautioned, "Beware of words—they are dangerous things."[12] And physicians' words are more dangerous than most. When you engage in diagnostics you need to be ever vigilant about your pronouncements because they have the potential to bring both order and chaos to the world of doctor and patient.

You can help temper the dangers associated with diagnostics by appreciating too what diagnostics is meant to achieve in a palliative care context. Diagnosis in palliative care is different than conventional acute care medicine. In palliative care one does not engage in diagnostics to promote a cure but rather to relieve the burdens of a progressive and terminal condition. Here diagnosis has comfort as its primary goal.

One of our medical students commented on how different this was from the prevailing ethos of acute care medicine. While working on the Pain and Palliative Care Service at Memorial Sloan-Kettering Cancer Center, she was amazed to observe that everything that was being done there diagnostically and therapeutically was *to make the patient more comfortable*.

This is a different mindset that you will need to consider as you think about diagnosis in palliative care. Here differential diagnosis is an exercise intimately related to realizing the goals of care. Your diagnostic reasoning may not be to realize a cure but to figure out *why* a patient has a certain pain syndrome or symptom complex. If you can determine that the pain in the patient's leg comes from metastatic bony lesions, you can intervene with local radiation therapy or systemic etidronate for pain relief. Here your diagnostics skills are being harnessed, *not to effect a cure*, but rather to bring the *proper* palliative care intervention to bear upon the patient's symptom burden. And it goes without saying that diagnostic precision for the achievement of palliation should be as sophisticated and rigorous as that in acute care settings.

Forced Prognostication and Patient Expectations

Prognosis		Comments:
> 6 mo	[ ]	_____
2 wk - 6mo	[ ]	_____
< 2 wk	[ ]	_____

Figure 9.2

Our consideration of goal setting continues with an effort at forced prognostication. Although we have addressed the difficulty of prognosis in Chapter 8, there is value in attempting prognostication when caring for patients near the end of life. Rarely will you find specific references to a patient's prognosis in the medical record, or hear a discussion of it on rounds until the very end of that person's life. Nonetheless, it is a good exercise to think about where the patient is on his disease trajectory. This can help better structure the goals of care and avoid misconstruals about potential outcomes. It can also help patients make plans and attend to professional and personal obligations.

The time frames offered above reflect both clinical perceptions and public policy. A life expectancy of six months is an important delineation. As we have noted in Chapter 7, a life expectancy of six months or less makes a patient eligible for hospice referral. In addition, a national survey of internists found that an overwhelming majority defined "terminal" as less than 6-months survival.[13]

Having noted this, it is still important to identify patients with a life-threatening illness with a life expectancy longer than six months. Because of our perceptions about terminal illness, such patients can fall prey to being seen exclusively in curative terms. And because of this, these patients are often treated in a manner that discounts palliation.

You might see this in a patient with advanced Alzheimer's disease who is physically in good health or a patient with aortic stenosis and cardiomyopathy who is not a surgical candidate. Both of these patients can be expected to have a life expectancy that can be counted in years, although each could have a symptom burden that could argue for palliative care.

Because of these perceptions about terminal illness, patients with a life-threatening disease but with a relatively longer life expectancy can easily be thought of in curative terms. The life-threatening nature of their illness can be denied because it is less imminent and they are at risk of being treated in a manner that discounts palliative care options. Such a situation might occur in a patient with Alzheimer's disease who is physically in good health or a patient with aortic stenosis and cardiomyopathy who is not a surgical candidate. Both of these patients have a life expectancy that can be counted in years although each may have a symptom burden that could argue for a palliative approach. When considering such patients it is important to be aware of prevailing perceptions about terminal illness lest patients be treated in a manner unbefitting their clinical and broader psychosocial needs.

The patient with an estimated prognosis of two weeks to six months should be thought of as a patient who is making a transition in expectations. At the same time, it is important to recognize that many of these patients are pursuing dual realities, accepting and denying death while living life.[14]

As they progress through this process their aspirations may change. Dr. David Kuhl in his book, *What Dying People Want*, has written eloquently about the authenticity that comes with the knowledge of a terminal condition.

The experience of learning about a terminal illness can propel someone into a search for a true self, a search for healing, for the courage to care for psychological wounds. It is the only way to live life to the fullest until one dies. One discards what's imitation and embraces what's real. This is a continuous process, which seems to move people from depression toward hope, through anxiety toward peace, and from despair toward integrity.[15]

A helpful way to think about this period of life is to help the dying live life to its fullest as defined by them, given the constraints of their illness and symptoms. Life becomes especially precious to patients when they know that they are facing finitude. Instead of using their valuable days and weeks attending clinic sessions for another round of therapy that may prove futile, patients may opt for palliation that minimizes their symptom burden and allows them to use their valuable time differently.

It is also important to know when patients have transitioned to a more imminent death and have a life expectancy of less than two weeks. This may be more obvious in patients with more "conventional" end of life trajectories such as cancer than those with congestive heart failure whose course might wax and wane.[16] In a retrospective review of deaths at our institution, patients with cancer and AIDs were far more likely to be identified as dying or have a DNR order than those with heart disease.[17]

Patients near the end of life, whose death is inevitable, need to be protected against the routine escalation of care that can accompany a growing symptom burden. For example, consider the patient with widely metastatic adenocarcinoma with involvement of the lung.[18] The patient is becoming increasingly dyspneic from Adult Respiratory Distress Syndrome. Previously the patient had expressed a desire to forgo resuscitation and signed a DNR order. As he gasps for air, a resident asks him if he would like to go on a breathing machine to make him more comfortable. With this as his only option, the patient agrees to mechanical ventilation, is intubated and whisked off to the ICU. Such are the routines of care in the acute care setting.

While mechanical ventilation is indeed one way to respond to the patient's air hunger, you need to protect your patients from routine therapeutic responses, like intubation, which are inconsistent with the patient's previously expressed preferences and ill-suited to an irreversible condition. Instead, you should think about more proportionate palliative approaches such as the use of intravenous morphine for air hunger.

Whatever the time frame, the essential point to thinking about prognosis is to have a sense of the time remaining. In this way, you can help your patients and their families plan for the inevitable and make the most of the time that is left.

Assessment of Capacity and the Refusal of Life-Sustaining Therapies

Patient Capacity:		Comments:
Yes [ ]	Variable [ ]	_____
No [ ]	Unclear [ ]	_____

Figure 9.3

Before continuing with the GCAT, we must know if the patient is "capable" of making decisions autonomously. As we discussed in Chapter 6, the patient's right to make decisions is protected as long as the patient has decision-making capacity. In cases where it is not clear if the patient is capacitated, a formal capacity assessment should be obtained through a psychiatry consult.[19] (See Chapter 10.) In those cases where capacity is unclear or variable, evaluation may be ongoing.

Again, it is important to appreciate that capacity can wax and wane. Patients may retain the ability to make some choices but be unable to make other more complex decisions. You must always be vigilant to the issue of capacity. At the end of life, the situation can be very fluid. Such patients are especially prone to delirium and changes in their mental status.[20] Depression can also alter the patient's decision-making abilities, sometimes meeting a rational standard but not an affective one.[21] At the end of life, patient decisions can also be affected by anxiety, medications, hypoxia, infection, or electrolyte disturbances. Every effort should be made to improve the decision-making ability of these patients, and to communicate with them during periods of lucidity. During these windows, it is important to elicit their preferences for end-of-life care. Patients who lack an advance directive should be asked to consider one, especially if it is expected that a subsequent loss of decision-making ability will be permanent.

In practice, the question of decision-making capacity often arises in the context of a treatment refusal. For example an elderly patient with a long history of atherosclerotic heart disease might refuse the cardiologist's recommendation for a cardiac catheterization to evaluate unstable angina. Up to this point the patient had been compliant with the doctor's recommendations. This refusal raises concerns that the patient has lost the ability to make judgments or is depressed. It is important to remember that a treatment refusal is not necessarily a sign of decisional incapacity just because a patient's choice goes against a physician's recommendation.[22]

Knowledge of Diagnosis and Prognosis

	Information			
	Yes	No	Unknown	Comments:
Patient aware of diagnosis	[ ]	[ ]	[ ]	_____
Patient aware of prognosis	[ ]	[ ]	[ ]	_____
Friend/Family/ Surrogate				
aware of diagnosis	[ ]	[ ]	[ ]	_____
aware of prognosis	[ ]	[ ]	[ ]	_____

Figure 9.4

In order to discuss matters effectively and sensitively with patients and surrogates, it is essential to establish how much they know about the diagnosis and prognosis. There can be huge gaps between what the clinician meant to say, or thinks was said to the patient, and what the patient understands. It is not at all unusual for physicians to write progress notes such as, "Discussed situation at length with patient and family," "Patient aware of poor prognosis," or "Discussed DNR with wife."[1] Colleagues reading these notes might assume that the patient or spouse knows the diagnosis and prognosis, but that is not a safe assumption.

In ethics case consultations, particularly futility disputes, we are often told by the patient or family member involved that although they have spoken with the doctor, the doctor never said anything about dying. The clinician may not have been clear in what was said, or the patient may be in denial and could not take in the bad news. In either case, this suggests that a starting point in formulating goals of care is knowing what the patient and surrogates know.

Consider the situation graphically displayed below:

Information			
	Yes	No	Unknown	Comments:
Patient aware of diagnosis	[X]	[ ]	[ ]	_____
Patient aware of prognosis	[ ]	[X]	[ ]	_____
Friend/Family/ Surrogate				
aware of diagnosis	[X]	[ ]	[ ]	_____
aware of prognosis	[X]	[ ]	[ ]	_____

Figure 9.5

A patient and family know the patient's diagnosis but only the family appreciates its gravity. This is a scenario that raises a number of questions that you will need to address. Why isn't the patient more fully informed? Did the physician fail to give a complete and full assessment of the situation? And if so, why does the family know? What does this say about family dynamics and modes of communication? Or, were they told about the prognosis but failed to accept its consequences? Has the family been trying to get the patient to be more realistic about expectations? Alternately, was the information given in a way the patient could not fully appreciate because of intervening anxiety, denial, or depression?

Viewing this scenario in tabular form helps to demonstrate the range of questions and possibilities that may flesh out this narrative. If you hope to work with this patient and family, you will need to understand why the patient and family know what they know, who told them the news and, most critically, what *meaning and emotional import* has been attached to the diagnostic and prognostic information. Although we think about diagnosis and prognosis in physiologic terms—and through the prism of our own life narratives—patients and families ascribe different meanings to these categories.

S. Kay Toombs emphasizes the importance that biography and perspective play in the worldview of patients and physicians. Physicians are often "an assigner of meaning to the illness," although this interpretation is derived from the doctor's own life experience and this may differ from that of the patient. Toombs suggests that making this perspectival bias explicit can

> prove invaluable in enabling the physician to begin the task of constructing a shared world of meaning with the patient. The doctor who monitors personal reactions and feelings towards the patient and the patient's illness, is better able to recognize and set aside any preconceived notions which may impede the ability to explore the meanings inherent in the patient's world. In this respect it is important to note that, in face-to-face contact with patients, physicians may come to experience illness as "frustrating," "boring," "interesting," "a limitation on one's capacities," "a challenge to one's expertise," and so forth. In other words, the physician's lived experience of the patient's illness is significantly different from the patient's lived experience of the patient's illness.[23]

Constructing a Shared World of Meaning with the Patient and Family

The first time you appreciate that your lived experience is different from your patient's is when you begin to know your patient. It happened to me when I was a third year medical student on the neurology service. I had been assigned a patient in his late forties dying of adenocarcinoma of the lung. He had metastatic disease, which had disseminated to his brain. Part of the tumor had been surgically resected from his occipital lobe. He had undergone radiation therapy, had a field cut, and was hemiplegic. I was instructed to give him chemotherapy three times a week through a special shunt connected to his cerebrospinal fluid.

Although I might now question the use of chemotherapy when a palliative care approach might be more fitting, as a student I accepted the mythic hope that the chemotherapy would bathe the tumor and retard its progress. Reflecting on the task now, I see it was a grim assignment that no on else wanted to do. He was dying and there wasn't much left to be done, so it was delegated to me, the medical student, the person with the least amount of experience, though this was a time of great significance for him.

Over time, we came to know each other. I learned that my patient had once enjoyed a successful career in business but that his rise to the top was cut short by alcoholism. He nearly lost everything but made a heroic comeback over the previous ten years. He stopped drinking, found new work, and married late in life to a wonderful woman who loved him dearly. He had finally found happiness and fulfillment. All of this was interrupted by the diagnosis of cancer.

As I administered the chemotherapy with sterile drapes covering his face, he told me he knew he was dying. He was very literate and recited from *Hamlet*. I recall the fenestrated drapes moving above his face as he recalled the lines and I slowly infused the methotrexate into his shunt. What he spoke from his deathbed has become ever more poignant to me now:

To die, to sleep—
No more, and by a sleep to say we end
The heartache and the thousand natural shocks
That flesh is heir to—'tis a consummation
Devoutly to be wished. To die to sleep.
To sleep, perchance to dream. Ay, there's the rub,
For in that sleep of death what dreams may come
When we have shuffled off this mortal coil
Must give us pause. There's the respect
That makes calamity of so long life
For who would bear the whips and scorns of time . . .[24]

He was glad that there was someone (albeit a medical student) to listen to him, even though I did not appreciate then that he might have been alluding to a desire to die, even suicide. It is ironic that as I write this twenty years later, I now realize—for the first time—that *I might have missed one of the very triggers* that I have asked you to consider. In retrospect, I take some consolation from the fact that I did in fact listen empathetically. This gave him an opportunity to share forgone hopes and current fears and to talk with someone.

But most of the time, he would ask about his wife and speak of his love for her. He told me of the financial arrangements he had made so that she would be comfortable after his death. He had set everything out carefully, although he never spoke with her about his financial planning. He voiced relief that she did not know he was dying. He did not want to inflict that kind of pain on someone he loved so much.

I said nothing. I knew differently. She had already asked me when he was going to die. All she really wanted was the opportunity to tell him just how much she loved him. She held back because she did not want to upset him *because he didn't know yet.*

As a medical student, it was difficult to watch them together. I knew they were aware that death was near but they *never* talked about it. They simply exchanged pleasantries when there was so much else they wanted to say. It reminded me of the film *The Pride of the Yankees* and the beneficent conspiracy of silence that enveloped Gary Cooper and Theresa Wright when Lou Gehrig was diagnosed with amyotrophic lateral sclerosis.[25] Both knew what this diagnosis meant but neither spoke a word of it to the other. Their silence was motivated by their deep love for each other and neither wanted to inflict pain.

Like *The Pride of The Yankees*, what I witnessed was a touching demonstration of love but also one of misplaced devotion. All I could see was a tragedy of mutual isolation. They only had so much time left together and they *needed* to talk.

The patient's wife once asked me in the hall if he knew that he was dying. It was an awkward situation. His attending was not around much because there was no hope and I was left to my own devices. So when she asked me if the patient knew, I simply said I didn't really know. It seemed wrong for me to betray the patient's trust or overstep the student's role. Better to get them to talk.

As the weeks passed he spoke more about his estate planning and all the arrangements he had made for his wife's financial security. I took this as an opening. "Wouldn't it be a good idea to tell her what you've done?" I never said that he should talk explicitly about dying. Instead, I sought to give voice to his own way of expressing his concerns about mortality and his wife's future. He dealt with his own mortality by seeking to secure his wife's financial future, a task with which he was professionally comfortable.

Given his concerns, I suggested that he speak with her about all the estate planning he had undertaken. Gently, I suggested that much of it could come to naught if she was not adequately informed now. I also spoke with her. "You know, he probably knows what's going on. And he'd really benefit from hearing what you have to say."

And then I waited to see what would happen. A couple of days passed. His condition worsened and the pleasantries continued. Then one morning I came back to the floor and they were in the room together *talking*. I also recall that they were holding hands.

Out of their silence came a wellspring of conversation. During the remaining six weeks of his life, they reaffirmed their love for each other. Where there was once isolation and distance there was now companionship, closeness and renewed intimacy. With a little prompting, they constructed a shared world of meaning, allowing for a peaceful death and easier bereavement for my patient and his beloved wife.

To usher people through a process of ending such conspiracies of silence may, in fact, be one of the most significant contributions we can make for patient and family at life's end. Fostering engagement can reduce suffering and isolation, which in turn allays the grief of the survivors.

Breaking Bad News

In attempting to determine what the patient does and does not know, you will encounter patients who need to be told their diagnosis and prognosis. Breaking bad news is difficult for even the most experienced of clinicians. It is even more challenging when you are in training and the patient is new to you. Indeed, a recent study of ethical conflicts encountered by house staff listed "telling the truth" as a leading cause of distress.[26]

If you find yourself in a situation where a patient needs to be told important life-altering information, you should first see whether there is a physician who has had an ongoing relationship with the patient. This can be therapeutic. A pre-existing doctor–patient relationship can help put the news into context and make it more credible. It is also a good preventative strategy. Bad news coming from an unknown and junior clinician can be discounted or more easily denied. It may also add to the suffering or sense of abandonment of the patient.

If you are called upon to break bad news, and you will be, it is important to be prepared. You will want to know about the information and think through its consequences and implications *before you start talking.* If at all possible, arrange your schedule so that you have time for the conversation and do not feel any additional pressure. If you are in the clinic, you might consider scheduling the appointment last so that breaking difficult news is the final task of the session and not the first one that must be confronted along with ten other patient visits. Before that visit, you should seek to prepare the patient for the *possibility* of disturbing news.

Consider the patient who you have sent for a colonoscopy to evaluate microcytic anemia and guiac positive stools. During the discussions about informed consent you will want to talk about the rationale for the test (to determine the source of bleeding and intercede early for a pre-malignant or malignant lesion). These potential risks and the benefits of early intervention ethically justify the lesser risks of endoscopy and so need to be disclosed as part of the consent process. Here the informed consent process not only provides patient authorization for the procedure, it also helps to prepare the patient for a possible adverse outcome, if spoken in a way which the patient truly understands what is being said. For most patients this will be reassuring, although it is very important to remain sensitive to those patients who will leap to the conclusion that they have cancer simply because you are looking to do this test.

You should suggest that a family member or friend join the patient when you reconvene to discuss the biopsy results. Plan this ahead of the procedure so that the patient does not think that it portends bad news. It is anxiety producing to call the day before your follow-up visit and say, "By the way, why don't you come into the office tomorrow with your wife." The patient will most certainly suspect bad news. It is better to arrange that family come to the follow-up visit ahead of time and make this your routine practice. If there is good news, the visit becomes an opportunity to celebrate. If not, the patient has some one there for support and to provide an extra set of ears.

You may counter that this is a lot of effort for a test that usually comes out okay. The odds of it being a benign polyp are significant so in all likelihood the outcome of the study will be innocent. You may be tempted to treat the procedure as a routine test and most of the time you will be correct. But in the event that the cause of the bleeding is potentially life-altering, it is important to be prepared and lay the foundation of what might be the beginning of the patient's end-of-life care. It is important to start the process with integrity, lest you lose the patient's trust and confidence as the disease progresses.[27]

Dr. Robert Buckman offers a helpful protocol for a breaking bad news approach turning to the practical aspects of the actual conversation.[28,29] Buckman suggests that the clinician first evaluate the setting in which the conversation will take place. One should be sure there is a comfortable place to sit eye-to-eye. If you consider sitting on the patient's bed, ask permission to do so. Hallways and hospital corridors are inappropriate places to have these conversations. Patients and families will be distracted and deprived privacy. Furthermore, the setting demeans the significance of these conversations. Find a meeting room and quiet space that provides a sanctuary from the usual hospital environment. This will improve the quality of the conversation and also show that you cared enough to plan ahead.

You should carefully consider the presence of the patient's family or friends and provide the patient the opportunity to be alone or supported by others. The patient's views may be constrained by others in the room or bolstered by their presence.

You want to be totally engaged with the patient. Dr. Jeremiah Barondess echoing Walsh McDermott's invocation of the Samaritan functions of the physician suggests that our role is "to counsel, to support, to create a genuine and relatively unhurried alliance, in addition to the equally important disease-based needs of our patients."[30] Practically, this means making good eye contact and conveying through body language that the patient has your full attention. Ask that the television and radio be turned off. Don't answer an e-mail on your Blackberry or allow your colleagues to interrupt you. Be empathic.

You might start the conversation by asking the bedridden patient if they are comfortable and adjust the bed or pillow. These gestures speak volumes to your concern and *if* the patient is uncomfortable it will have helped make it possible for them to attend to what you have to say. Touch may also be an important feature of compassion, if culturally appropriate, and if the gesture is an appropriate hand on the shoulder or arm.

Provide the patient with the information about the test result and provide direction while still giving the patient the opportunity to make her own choices. This is a difficult balance to achieve. If you are too open-ended with the patient, she may feel that you are uncertain about next steps and may question your competence. This will add to the patient's anxiety. Too much direction can impede the patient's ability to direct his or her own care.

Use a variety of listening strategies—open-ended questions, periods of silence, and nonverbal encouragement for the patient to speak—to find the right balance for each particular patient. To begin, you need to ascertain the patient's perception of her condition and its seriousness. An innocent question might be, "Did Dr. Smith speak with you after the colonoscopy?" This is an important starting point because you do not know *if she knows* that a polyp was found and that biopsy was taken. She may assume that because she wasn't told about a biopsy it hadn't happened. She's expecting that you will tell her that everything is just fine. Or, she might have been told about a biopsy while she was still sedated and forgotten the conversation.

Either scenario points to why it is important to start with what the patient already knows, or is prepared to acknowledge. Follow this step by asking if the patient is interested in knowing more. If the patient desires more information, you should begin with the patient's state of knowledge. In our example, you might report that a polyp was removed and then provide the biopsy results.

Information should be given in language that is appropriate to the patient's level of understanding. By asking questions and listening to her choice of words you will gain an understanding of her language abilities and comprehension. Avoid jargon and technical terms. Speak in small and digestible chunks. Periodically, pause to confirm that the patient is following you: "Do you have any questions about this?" or "I want to be sure that I have been clear. Could you share with me your understanding of the test results?"

You will be amazed how often you have been misunderstood or misconstrued, even when you were sure that you had been perfectly clear! Asking these open-ended questions may seem a bit patronizing but is really in the patient's best interest. Clarifying misconceptions can be very reassuring and help prevent unrealistic expectations later in the course of an illness. It also shows that you care enough to be sure the patient understands the results and their implications.

If the news is bad, it is critical to give the patient some time to incorporate what has been heard and to provide reassurance. You should acknowledge and explore the patient's emotional response to the news. Be sensitive to the patient's affect and respond to it. This may be accomplished by statements of empathy, "I sense you're disappointed that we found a cancerous polyp. But this can be treated."

When patients hear the word "cancer" most shut down and look inward pondering their own mortality. A detailed discussion of colon cancer staging and the fact that you think that this is an early lesion will be lost to the patient. If the patient asks for more information, provide it. But in most cases it is better to be directive and lay out a plan in conjunction with the patient. In this case, it might be to obtain a CAT scan and a referral to a surgeon. Or it might be to ask the patient if they would like to return later to continue or repeat the conversation, perhaps with another family member present.

When a consensus is reached regarding how to proceed, briefly summarize what was discussed, ask if there are any other questions, and set up your next appointment. A revisit in a couple of days is important to set a time frame and to provide a structure for your continued conversations with the patient.

Perhaps the most important thing you can do as a physician is to use the opportunity to reassert your fidelity to the patient. Your patient is scared and embarking on a voyage she has never taken. Above all she doesn't want to be abandoned by you. After all, you have demonstrated skill and care in helping to make the diagnosis. She trusts you and needs your continued help. Be empathic and supportive. If the patient is upset you might say: "I know this is rough, but we'll *get through this together*." Alternately, you can say, "I want you to know that I am committed to participate in your care regardless of the outcome." Although you may hesitate to offer that cliche, an affirmation of your on-going commitment to the patient needs to be shared.

The Therapeutic Exception

In Chapter 2, we recounted the relationship of truth telling to the ethics of self-determination and the doctrine of informed consent. Simply put, for patients to be autonomous they need to have relevant information to make medical decisions. In American medical practice, disclosure of this information is the norm. But there are exceptions when the truth is withheld under the rubric of what is called the *therapeutic exception*. As its name would imply, invoking the exception, is a departure from the general norm to disclose the truth. Exceptional circumstances are needed for a physician to invoke his therapeutic *privilege* and withhold the truth. It is estimated that this privilege is invoked in less than 5 percent of cases involving disclosure of information.

The therapeutic exception is invoked when disclosure would be disproportionately dangerous or burdensome. An example might be disclosing a malignant biopsy to a patient who is hospitalized for suicidality. Here the benefits of disclosure are outweighed by the risks of providing a suicidal patient information that might further imperil his well-being.

An alternate rationale for withholding the truth might be the case of the recently immigrated patient from another country where truth telling is not the norm. North American medical ethics, as we have seen in Chapters 2 and 3, places a premium on patient self-determination through the vehicle of informed consent. But other cultures have differing norms. One study of truth-telling norms among European-Americans, African-Americans, Mexican-Americans, and Korean-Americans indicated that each placed a different value on disclosure.[31] European-Americans and African-Americans valued being informed to put their financial or spiritual affairs in order. Korean-Americans, in contrast, were less interested in being informed, preferring to save face. Mexican-American respondents staked out an intermediate position. Such differences are important to appreciate because they may lead to differing views about the use of life-sustaining therapies at the end of life.[32]

I recall one elderly Chinese patient who was being evaluated for epigastric pain who, when given the opportunity to know a diagnosis, opted not to know. Although cognitively intact, when asked if she would like to know more about her condition, she responded in Chinese, "my memory is very weak; you should speak to my son." This was her way of saving face and delegating authority to a family member, in line with her cultural tradition.

Given the risks associated with idiosyncratic judgments about withholding the truth, in most clinical settings this determination requires the agreement of two physicians—and possibly the involvement of an ethics committee—to determine that the sharing of information would be disproportionate and that the invocation of the therapeutic exception is warranted. This safeguard is in place to avoid unilateral decisions on the part of physicians to withhold disturbing news.

Articulated Preferences for End-of-Life Care

Preferences Regarding Life-Sustaining Therapy:			
	Yes	No	Unknown
DNR	[ ]	[ ]	[ ]
Comments: _____			
Advance Directive	[ ]	[ ]	[ ]
_____			
Health Care Proxy:	[ ]	[ ]	[ ]
_____			
Living Will:	[ ]	[ ]	[ ]
_____			
Name: _____			
Phone: _____			

Figure 9.6

DNR orders and advance directives were discussed at length in Chapter 7. This section is geared to helping you collect this important information. This may seem like a trivial or clerical task but, remarkably, over 50 percent of physicians in the SUPPORT study on end of life care *did not know* that their patients had a DNR order.[33] If you want to respect the choices that patients make for care near the end of life, you need to be aware of their preferences.

Unfortunately, DNR orders and Advance Directives do not travel well. Information received from a previous site of care may not be legible, comprehensive, or easily incorporated into the format used by the receiving facility or agency. It is a sad commentary on our priorities that dying patients who are transferred from one institution to another are more likely to arrive with their liver function studies than documentation outlining their preferences for end-of-life care. When patients are transferred, it is important to look for these documents and call the referring institution to guide decision making.

Depending on geographic location, emergency medical services may not honor a DNR order while a patient is being transported. This can lead to discontinuity of care from one venue to the next and have patients receiving life-sustaining intervention against their wishes.[34] This is remedied in many states through portable DNR statutes that allow for the transfer of DNR orders from one institution to another and for DNR orders in the home.[35]

Patients who do arrive with a DNR order from another institution are not automatically DNR upon admission. The prior order generally needs to be assessed and reissued by the attending physician after evaluation of the patient. Though the patient's DNR order is contingent until the directive is reauthorized for the hospital setting, the patient's prior intentions can be immensely helpful in guiding future decisions about resuscitation.[36]

DNR in the OR

One particular DNR scenario calls out for special mention—when a patient with a pre-existing DNR order requires surgery. Many clinicians feel strongly that DNR orders should be unilaterally suspended when a patient is taken for surgery.[37] They argue that it is ethically untenable for a patient to have surgery and remain DNR because the very act of inducing anesthesia and operating can cause the patient to have a cardiac arrest. Furthermore, it is difficult to know in the operating room whether you are letting nature takes its course and letting a patient die or if the cause of the arrest is because of a medical intervention. Because these arrests may be caused by a clinical intervention, critics of DNR orders in the operative setting argue that they should be reversed. They maintain that the mandate for resuscitation in the OR is even stronger because the likelihood of success is greater when the patient has a witnessed arrest in a controlled setting and is already intubated.[38] One large study reported a 65 percent survival rate for intra-operative arrests and a 92 percent rate if they were anesthesia related.[39] Another older study found that the chances of survival were ten times higher if an arrest occurred while under anesthesia than if it happened on a medical floor.[40]

These are good arguments, but they are technical ones. Although the likelihood of success is something that patients or their surrogate decision makers should know when making a judgment about resuscitation, the decision regarding resuscitation should be theirs as an expression of the patient's self-determination. (See Chapters 1–3.) The centrality of patient or surrogate choice is ensconced in law. For example, New York's DNR Law provides that no clinician may prohibit issuance of a DNR order as a precondition for receiving health care services such as surgery. According to state law, DNR orders can only be suspended with the permission of the patient, agent, or surrogate.[41]

But as we recognize the centrality of patient autonomy in these choices, we are also struck by the ethical paradox of operating on patients who have articulated a preference to be left alone. In a sense these patients are asking you "to do something (operate) but leave me alone (don't resuscitate)." This intersection of the negative right to be left alone and the positive entitlement to have something done is paradoxical *unless both actions are consistent with a common goal of care.*

The need for a *coherence of goals* of care becomes clear if we consider two operative procedures. Consider a patient who consents to a coronary artery bypass and another who needs a diverting colostomy for obstructing colon cancer. Let's imagine that both want to go to the OR with a DNR order in place.

The first patient's goals of care are internally inconsistent because cardioplegia, that is cardiac arrest, is necessary for the bypassing of the coronary arteries. Here a desire to have the procedure and be DNR *are mutually exclusive and illogical.*

But in the second case, they are not. There is a logic to retaining a DNR order when a patient goes for a diverting colostomy. Here the patient with advanced cancer and intractable pain is asking to have a *palliative* procedure for symptom relief. His goal is comfort and not life-prolongation. He had been DNR prior to surgery and wants to maintain this designation. From his point of view, it does not really matter whether he dies on the floor or in the operating room.

Although taking any patient to the operating room with a DNR order seems to be counter-intuitive, it can be appropriate when we consider surgery as a palliative rather than a curative intervention. And if we view these surgical procedures as a palliative intervention, then we need to maintain the patient's dual prerogatives of pain relief and the right to refuse life-sustaining therapy. Forcing patients to accept resuscitation to obtain a palliative procedure is ethically untenable because we are compelling patients to give up their negative right to be left as a precondition for pain-relieving surgery.[42]

Ideally, the best way to handle these potential dilemmas is to prevent them. Clarifying the goals of care in anticipation of surgery can do this. In this regard we have guidance from a position statement from the American College of Surgeons. They recommend that patients or their surrogates have an opportunity to review preexisting DNR orders prior to surgery as part of the informed consent process. This process of "required reconsideration" is worth quoting at length.

> Policies that lead either to the automatic enforcement of all DNR orders and requests or to disregarding of automatic cancellation of such orders and requests during the operation and the recovery period may not sufficiently address a patient's right to self-determination. An institutional policy of automatic cancellation of the DNR status in cases where a surgical procedure is to be carried out removes the patient from appropriate participation in decision making. Automatic enforcement without discussion and clarification may lead to inappropriate peri-operative and anesthetic management. The best approach is a policy of "required reconsideration" of previous advance directives. The patient and the physicians who will be responsible for the patient's care should discuss the new risks and the approach to potential life threatening problems during the peri-operative period.[43]

The Elusive Advance Directive

In Chapter 7, we reviewed the types of advance directives and their relative strengths. This section will address how advance care planning unfolds in clinical practice.

The first question to consider when a patient lacks capacity is whether any written or verbal directions exist. Did the patient complete an advance directive? If it is a Health Care Proxy, who did the patient designate as the agent, and how can that person be reached? If the advance directive is a Living Will, what does it say about preferences related to end-of-life care? Is there any other evidence of the patient's wishes? Has the patient discussed them with staff members or family? In the absence of a written directive, information should be sought from the patient's family, significant others, personal physician, clergyman, and others to gain more knowledge of the patient's values and wishes.

Sometimes you will really need to be a sleuth to find the information you will need. I recall one case brought to the ethics consultation service when we were asked to assist with the case of a woman in her 90s who had had coronary artery bypass surgery. She had been in the hospital for several months and she could never be sustained for more than a few days at a time off the ventilator. Her course had also been complicated by a sternal wound infection.

The team approached the patient's sister to ascertain any prior wishes regarding the withdrawal of life-sustaining therapy. The sister, in her late 80s with some mild memory deficits, could not recall any prior conversation. There was no written advance directive.

The ethics consultation team was asked to get involved and we determined that the patient had been initially cared for in the general medical clinic. She had been referred to the cardiology service by them. Over time, as her care grew more complex, she moved from one clinical service to the next from Medicine to the CCU to Cardiothoracic Surgery and the Cardiology Consult Service. She was no longer being followed by Medicine.

The ethics consultation team went back to the outpatient medical record in the General Medicine Clinic. A resident had written a note that he had discussed advance directives with the patient but there was no completed advance directive in the chart. We wondered whether the patient had said anything to the resident that might guide decision making. We tracked the resident down. He was working as a flight surgeon in the Air Force on the West Coast and he recalled the patient and the conversation. They had talked about advance care planning. The patient said she did not want to be maintained on machines. She neither completed an advance directive nor designated her sister as her health care proxy because she did not want to burden her. Because the patient did not formally fill out the required form, the resident thought that no advance care planning had occurred and never documented the content of the conversation, only that he had raised the issue. But this was an error. She had articulated preferences; she simply had not filled out the form.

When we spoke to the patient's sister about this conversation with the former resident, she remembered him and recalled the content of the conversation. "Oh, yes, she said she never wanted to be on machines." So informed, a decision was made to withdraw life-sustaining therapy. The patient died peacefully after a fitful battle with protracted heart disease.

This vignette has two messages. First, it is critical to document patient preferences even when the patient has not filled out the advance directive form. What is verbally said has moral and legal standing and can direct care. The second point is to look carefully for information about preferences, especially in settings that are prone to discontinuity of care.

Placing the Patient in Context

Family Support:			
	Yes	No	Unknown
Does patient have friends/family	[ ]	[ ]	[ ]
Involved Family	[ ]	[ ]	[ ]
Identified Spokesperson(s): _____			
Relationship: _____			
Family preferences: _____			
Psychosocial issues: _____			
Cultural issues: _____			
Discussion with Patient/Family: _____			

Figure 9.7

Family Dynamics

Commenting upon the role of families in futility disputes, the philosopher James Lindenmann Nelson poignantly reminds us that it is within the intimate relationships of family and deep friendship that we construct ourselves.[44,45] These relationships shape our core values and accommodate our most important needs. The love and support of family* can be an important balm and intimates can helpfully represent the patient when decisional incapacity occurs. For all these reasons, families need to be taken seriously and given proper deference.

---

*Family is broadly defined here including biological and *chosen* family, close friends and other intimates.

Beyond their moral standing, families have tremendous instrumental value in providing care to the patient. It is hard to know a patient without knowing the family. Family members can help provide insight and perspective. Who is this person, beyond the hospital and their disease? Who are the important people in the patient's life, those who love, support or depend on him? What should you know about those relationships in order to better understand and provide compassionate care? What does the family want you to know about the patient, and what do they think about future care? What are their worries and how are they conveyed to *or* withheld from the patient?

Although your primary ethical allegiance is to the patient, both patient and the family should be the object of your ministrations. To focus on the patient at the exclusion of the family is to discount the burdens and consequences of terminal illness that *metastasize* beyond the patient. Illness impacts upon the psychological and physical health of fellow family members and their economic well-being. Rates of depression soar when there is serious illness in the family and serious illness in one member of the family predisposes close family members to own their own illnesses. To care for the patient, it is imperative to support those who love and care for the patient.

The interdependence of patient and family runs counter to notions of the doctor–patient dyad, but in fact that construction is too simplistic. For all these reasons, in hospice care there is a saying that the *unit of care is the family*. This is a valuable admonition that becomes increasingly important when you have to work with the patient's surrogates.

There are a number of things you can do to create an alliance with the patient's family and intimates. It is best if you have a pre-existing relationship before confronting a crisis. As we have noted in Chapter 6, a good doctor–patient relationship does not necessarily translate into one between doctor and family, especially if you are meeting the family after the patient has deteriorated and can not speak for herself. In that situation, there may be a tendency for family members to express their anxiety and concern by being suspicious about you and your expertise. Afterall, the backdrop for your encounter is bad news and you are its messenger.

Whether or not you are meeting family members for the first time or just seeing them again, you will want to provide them with timely updates and be accessible. Let them know that you are available and that there are "no dumb questions," except for the ones that are not asked. If they know that you can be reached, chances are they will only call you when there is a true need. If they are uncertain about your accessibility, they may call to test you. So be available. Go out of your way to make a call or stop by. The small amount of time expended in these gestures can demonstrate that you care and that your concern transcends the merely physiologic components of care. A little bit of preventive outreach can be extremely important in relationship building.

When dealing with a large family you will want to identify a spokesman for the entire family when the patient can not speak for him or herself. This should be a designated surrogate or the patient's next of kin—the person to whom you would turn normally to discuss treatment options. While you should be available for family meetings when a major decision is being made or a transition is being negotiated, it is best to speak to one person who will communicate what you have said to other family members. Multiple conversations with different family members can become very time consuming and can lead to miscommunication and discord.

The Symbionic Family

Most families will work together for the good of the patient and these families will work with you too. In others, the relationships will have been marred by years of conflict, dysfunction, distrust, or mental illness. These families will present challenges because of the additional stress associated with facing death.

The first bit of advice to be offered is to be aware of your frustration. You need to accept that you will not be able to fix in death that which has always been dysfunctional in life. Your task should simply be to help the family achieve the best death possible given the circumstances. You should seek to avoid adding to any additional stress by errors in communication or perceived indifference.

Though you would not willingly miscommunicate or seem indifferent to the needs of patients and families, the dysfunctional family dynamic will try to bring the worst out of you. You may become frustrated and angry and deviate from your usual practice patterns. Instead of striving to be of more help to a needy family, you may find yourself disappointed by what you failed to do or by errors that you would not normally make such as becoming angry with a demanding family member. Instead of engaging in self-reproach, it is more productive to understand which situations and family dynamics conjure up anger within you. In this way you can use your counter-transference as a diagnostic tool that can lead you to avoid iatrogenesis and provide better care.

Let us turn to a particularly challenging family scenario that we have not seen described in the literature but that our ethics case consultation service has encountered. For lack of a better descriptor, we call these families symbionic. A symbion is an organism that is melded with another and highly enmeshed with another. Psychic boundaries are blurred and it is hard to know where the needs, interests, and desires of one begins and the other ends.

Some of our most difficult cases involving families have been ones marked by a symbionic relationship: an elderly parent (usually a widowed mother) being attended to by a socially isolated child (generally a daughter) whose life has centered on the needs of a chronically ill parent. The two have created a world together marked by doctor visits, home care, and social isolation for both mother and daughter.

Until crisis strikes, theirs is a workable, though hardly optimal, strategy. A dutiful daughter selflessly gives up the possibility of friends, family, and independence to care for an ailing parent. But when the parent becomes ill and is facing death, the utility of the arrangement becomes suspect. Faced with the prospect of losing the only person in the world who matters to her, the daughter clings to her mother. This translates into spending hours on end at the bedside refusing to leave the hospital, compulsively keeping notes of every medication that is given down to the number of stool softeners. Or she might ask the doctors to give her ninety-year-old mother less pain medication so that they can talk, even though the record shows that the patient's dementia has made meaningful communication impossible for a decade.

Children can also be the objects of a symbionic relationship. In this dynamic, we have encountered adult children who have been unable to live independently and who have remained under a parental gaze that derives benefit from the continuation of the child's dependency.

We have seen a pattern in which the healthier symbion fails to accept the recommendations of the treating team and often fails to make any decisions at all. They often have *conflicting and inconsistent* goals of care for their loved one. They desperately want them to survive and therefore want everything to be done *but* at the same time refuse procedures that might be life-saving. Try as you might to get at the roots of the ambivalence, you are unable to use logic or emotion to expose the inconsistency of their wishes. This is more than the usual family ambivalence, fear, or confusion about the medical facts that generally are receptive to negotiation and compromise. Symbions are different. They are paralyzed by the prospect of making any decision because they are so frightened about making a bad choice about someone who literally is the world to them. Generally this means that aggressive care continues by default.

When you care for such patients you will likely be frustrated because you believe that the provision of aggressive care in hopeless situations is pointless and unethical. You hate to see the patient suffer especially when there is little hope that any burdens associated with treatment might result in cure or improvement. You are frustrated that your efforts at mediation fail and that your attempts at logic are cleverly rebuffed through arguments that are deeply flawed.

Work to harness your frustration and counter-transference because your feelings will only cause parent and child to further enmesh themselves into each other's life. Acknowledge their difficulty in facing death and empathically appreciate that the loss of their loved one means the loss of everything, including the loss of their way of life. Their years of sacrifice will come to an end and they will be fundamentally alone and angry at being abandoned. This anger may be directed at you and the care team.

Unfortunately, we do not have sage advice on how to resolve the dilemmas that will surely evolve out of symbiosis. Seek to identify this dynamic early so as not to make matters even more difficult and ask for the assistance of the consultation liaison psychiatrist. In our experience the psychiatrist can be helpful in setting up boundaries between the patient and symbion. This separation can make it easier to deal with each of them and help disentangle the potentially destructive components of the relationship while maintaining its constructive elements.

Cultural Issues: Religious Objections to Brain Death

When speaking of families we also need to appreciate the broader cultural context within which families operate. From whatever culture we hail, most of the time we will be providing care to someone who is in some way different from ourselves if we consider the variables of race, ethnicity, religion, class, and socioeconomic status. Each of these determinants can inform the clinical encounter and influence decisions near the end of life.[46,47]

Practically, an important issue is being sure that you are communicating adequately, especially if there are language barriers. Patients and families are at a tremendous disadvantage when they have to confront terminal illness as well as a foreign language admixed with the technical jargon of medicine.[48] You have an ethical obligation to ensure adequate translation services for your patients and families. This means more than translation by a relative who might not convey the truth to the patient or the ad hoc translation services of an unqualified staff member whose fluency or accuracy might be suspect, missing the subtleties of interpretation.[49] or whose involvement might be viewed as a breach of confidentiality by patient or family.[50]

Whatever background you bring to the patient's bedside, you will need to build a doctor–patient–family relationship. To that end, you will need to consider how to build bridges across cultures that will support and sustain the clinical transaction. The goal here should not be utopian understanding between varying cultures. If we aim that high, we will uniformly fail. Instead, we need to be more realistic and avoid reaching for this illusion of perfect universalism. Better to reach for an approximation of shared understanding that will promote discourse and civility when our collective diversity comes together in the clinical setting.[51]

There is perhaps no case that stresses pluralism and respect for diversity more than one involving a religious or moral objection to the declaration of death. Most readers will not encounter such cases because you are not in states that sanction an objection to brain death determinations. New York and New Jersey are the exception. Nonetheless, brain death objections are worth considering because lessons can be learned that will help you address other cross-cultural challenges in palliative care.

New York State, because of its religious diversity—most notably its Orthodox Jewish and Fundamentalist Christian populations—developed a policy on brain death determinations that allows for an objection to a brain death determination of death on religious or moral grounds. State policy requires "a procedure for the reasonable accommodation of the individual's religious or moral objection to the determination as expressed by the individual, or by the next of kin or other person closest to the individual." [52] A similar policy exists in New Jersey.

> The death of an individual shall not be declared upon the basis of neurological criteria . . . when the licensed physician authorized to declare death, has reason to believe . . . that such a declaration would violate the personal religious beliefs of the individual. In these cases, death shall be declared, and the time of death fixed, solely upon the basis of cardio-pulmonary criteria. [53]

In practice this means that patients who are legally dead under the Uniform Determination of Death Act accepted by 48 states,[54] can not be pronounced dead in New York or New Jersey if that determination violates religious beliefs. This accommodation of religious beliefs, in our region, provides the backdrop for the case of an Orthodox Hassidic Jewish patient who had herniated from an advanced brain tumor. An ethics consultation was requested when it appeared that the patient had become brain dead. The patient did not breathe when a preliminary apnea test was performed and this finding suggested whole brain death—the death of both cortex and brain stem functions. It did not confirm the diagnosis of brain death then because the prevailing legal norm for brain death required a second apnea test before a declaration of brain death could be made.

The patient's relative, after learning of the first apnea test, refused a second study and refused to leave the patient's bedside. She interposed herself between the doctors and the patient. She would have had to have been physically removed in order to perform the "confirmatory" study. And for added tension, all of this occurred on the eve of the Jewish High Holiday season.

As you might imagine, this was a potentially volatile situation. Theocentric and scientifically informed worldviews were being brought together in close proximity by tragic circumstances and conflict seemed inevitable. Many on the staff felt that they "were treating a corpse" and that all due deference to pluralism should not oblige them to that task. And beyond that there was anger—a reflection of staff counter-transference.[55] Difference was challenging their expertise, a scientific worldview internalized as an acceptance of the brain death definition, and their secularist identification.

How should this cultural clash be addressed? When cultures intersect, it is best to try and build trust and engage in a negotiation. In this case, we used the ambiguity of the medical facts as an opportunity for negotiation. Although there was a strong suspicion the patient was brain dead, the lack of a second apnea test did not make him *legally* brain dead. This diagnostic nuance provided an opportunity to gather more facts and begin a narrative journey to transform principled differences into resolvable disputes.

A first task is to examine your own worldview. Although clinicians take the definition of brain death as a given, a consideration of its origins reveals that this diagnosis is a *human construct* introduced in the Harvard Criteria in 1968[56] as a means to retrieve organs for transplantation. It is a concept that is ensconced in the law but has been more recently open to philosophical critique.[57,58] These facts can allow you to better appreciate the perspective of those who might object to the criteria. Ultimately they can help you appreciate that there is often a range of reasonable moral choices. None of us has moral—or scientific—certitude.

Although these reflections may still lead you to continue to equate brain death with the cessation of cardio-pulmonary function, they do provide an *opening* for the serious engagement of other perspectives. Part of that task is to explore that patient's cultural or religious tradition and to familiarize oneself with the general norms that might be relevant to the particulars of a case.

This can be done in two complementary ways. The first is by expanding the dyad and bringing in cultural intermediaries from the same group or tradition who can assist in guiding the deliberations and in the negotiation process. These individuals might be coreligionists or members of the same ethnic group who work in the health care setting and have a foot in both worlds. They can help translate the views of those involved in a dispute either literally or figuratively and provide the requisite trust needed for the discussion of delicate issues.

The second strategy is to be sure that the conflict is real and reflective of the groups' actual religious practices.[59] In this case, it would be wrong to assume that all Orthodox Jews reject brain death. Some Orthodox Jews accept brain death as if it were a physiologic decapitation[60] akin to a story in Talmud when an individual was decapitated by a tree. Although his heart was still beating, he was considered dead because the heart and the body could not be sustained without the head. Although the family depicted in this case were not of the sect that accepted brain death, it would have been grossly inattentive to fail to note differences *within* the tradition.

Again, it is critical to stress that when encountering difference, it is important to recognize that traditions are not monolithic and that there are a diversity of interpretations and views within a community. If we had stereotyped their beliefs, we would have done this family a disservice and perpetuated a difference that might not have existed. Knowledge of the family's cultural traditions also allows you to distinguish a religious or moral objection from responses that are more reflective of sadness and grief, that of relatives grieving for a lost loved one and not wanting to let go.

With the stage set in this way, we had a number of fruitful meetings with Rabbinic representatives of the family. In those meetings we sought to identify the range of moral considerations that might be common to our secular approach and their religiously informed view of the clinical situation. Assisted by cultural intermediaries, we mutually agreed *to abandon the divisive question of whether the patient was dead.* This was not a resolvable question. Though it started as the most important of considerations, it had in fact become a distraction. Instead we sought to reframe the problem pragmatically, drawing upon Jewish sources.

In this approach, we sought to move beyond a dispute over the moral meaning of brain death. We asked how Jewish law would interpret the conflicting mandates to preserve life but not prolong the dying process. Instead of struggling over a definition of brain death, we engaged the observant family, on their own terms, in the moral dilemma posed by a patient's illness.[61]

Our interventions helped to de-escalate a potentially volatile situation and fostered a dialogue across a religious and cultural divide. We negotiated a plan acceptable to both parties and withdrew some elements of ICU care. The patient ultimately suffered a cardio-pulmonary arrest and succumbed.

Although the case was not decided in accord with a secular or religious framework, a compromise was mediated through careful cultivation of the narrative and trust. Although this could be seen as a failure, it is more profitable to view it as a successful, albeit tragic, encounter of two differing worldviews.

And this is something that you should relish, the opportunity to know another culture and worldview from a privileged perspective. If seen in this way, differing worldviews will not be annoyance but a rewarding part of your professional life.

Assessing Symptoms

Pain and Symptom Inventory:			
Symptom:	Yes	No	Treated/Response:
Pain	[ ]	[ ]	_____
Anxiety	[ ]	[ ]	_____
Depression	[ ]	[ ]	_____
Cognitive Dysfunction	[ ]	[ ]	_____
Dyspnea	[ ]	[ ]	_____
Diarrhea	[ ]	[ ]	_____
Nausea/Vomiting	[ ]	[ ]	_____
Constipation	[ ]	[ ]	_____
Other Suffering	[ ]	[ ]	_____
Specify: _____			

Figure 9.8

It is important to comprehensively take stock of the patient's symptom burden. This assessment can help inform the goals of care and lead to enhanced patient comfort. This list is here to remind you to be comprehensive in your evaluation.

It is beyond our scope to describe each of these symptoms in detail. The goal here is to describe the kinds of data and information that you should seek out in your evaluation when assessing current symptoms and contemplating their mitigation. In this, you might be assisted by a framework offered by the Palliative Education Assessment Tool (PEAT) designed to improve the development of medical school curricula in palliative care and clinical ethics,[62,63] from which the following exhibits are excerpted. (See Exhibits 9-1, 9-2, 9-3.) Exhibit 9-1 delineates the issues that should inform your understanding of pain and pain management, including its public health dimensions, basic science aspects, and clinical therapies.

Exhibit 9-1 Pain

A. Epidemiology of pain and significance (i.e., public health view on pain at EOL for pts. and populations).

B. Barriers to adequate pain management (professional, political or economic, i.e., attitudes toward opioids, addiction, restrictive regulations, inadequate knowledge on the part of physicians, etc.)

C. Neurobiology of pain (i.e., pathophysiology of pain)

D. Pain characteristics (i.e., frequency, intensity, site, quality, triggers, acute/chronic, etc.)

E. Disease specific pain syndromes (i.e., cancer and AIDS related pain syndromes, etc.)

F. Pain-related history & physical exam (i.e., focused H&P to evaluate pain)

G. Complementary therapy history (e.g., elucidate patient's use of complementary therapies for pain such as acupuncture)

H. Diagnostic assessment of pain (i.e., ability to formulate differential diagnosis re: etiology/sources of pain, etc.)

I. Non-opioid pharmacologic management of pain (i.e., use of non-opioids, etc.)

J. Use of opioids (i.e., WHO analgesic ladder, tolerance, dependence, addiction, therapies, drug conversions, route of administration, dosing, etc.)

K. Non-pharmacologic management of pain (i.e., surgery, physical therapy, etc.)

From: Meekin SA, Klein JE, Fleischman AR, and Fins JJ. Development of a Palliative Education Assessment Tool for Medical Student Education. *Academic Medicine* 75(10)(2000):986–992.

It is also important to consider the scope of neuropsychological conditions that can influence patient care at the end of life. Exhibit 9-2 details the range of topics that may be relevant to your patients, including the epidemiology, neurobiology, and clinical presentation of symptoms ranging from agitation to delirium. It also points to therapeutic issues that are relevant to management of these symptom complexes.

Exhibit 9-2 Neuropsychologic Symptoms
(agitation, depression, delirium, dementia, etc.
and other mental status changes, as well as
psychological distress)

A. Epidemiology and significance (i.e., prevalence of depression at EOL)

B. Neurobiology of symptoms (i.e., agitation, depression, delirium, dementia, etc.)

C. Symptoms as complications of therapy (i.e., changes in mental status, i.e., sedation from opioids, etc.)

D. Disease specific neuropsych symptoms (i.e., influence of underlying disease on mental status, personality changes from frontal lobe tumor or AIDS related dementia, etc.)

E. Neuropsych symptom history & physical exam (i.e., mental status and directed physical exam, etc.)

F. Complementary therapy history (e.g., use of agents by patients for depression, i.e., St. John's Wort, etc.)
G. Diagnostic assessment of neuropsych syndromes (ability to formulate differential diagnosis using DSM IV)
H. Counseling/Psychotherapeutic
I. Pharmacologic management (i.e., treatment of depression with tricyclics and SSRIs, use of psychostimulants with opioids, etc.)
J. Other management strategies (i.e., acupuncture, complementary therapies, etc.)
K. Efficacy of neuropsych management (and ability to assess and revise treatment plan, i.e., adjust from one antidepressant class to another due to inefficacy).

From: Meekin SA, Klein JE, Fleischman AR, and Fins JJ. Development of a Palliative Education Assessment Tool for Medical Student Education. *Academic Medicine* 75(10)(2000):986–992.

Symptoms at the end of life are not limited to pain or the neuropsychological. Exhibit 9-3 outlines a strategy to comprehensively consider burdensome somatic symptoms, their diagnosis, and management.

Exhibit 9-3   Other Symptoms (i.e., dyspnea, nausea/ vomiting, constipation, diarrhea, pruritis, etc.)

A. Epidemiology and its significance
B. Pathophysiology of non-pain symptoms (i.e., pruritis in hepatobiliary disease, etc.)
C. Disease specific syndromes (i.e., AIDS related diarrhea, wasting and wt. loss in cancer, dyspnea in advanced lung disease, etc.)
D. Symptoms as complications of therapy (i.e., constipation from opioids, parathesias from chemotherapy, etc.)
E. Symptom history & physical exam (i.e., focused H&P to evaluate other symptoms)

F. Complementary therapy history (e.g., elucidate patient's use of complementary therapies for other symptoms)

G. Diagnostic assessment of non-pain syndromes (ability to formulate differential diagnosis regarding etiology/sources of other symptoms)

H. Pharmacologic management (i.e., laxatives for constipation, bronchodialators for respiratory compromise, etc.)

I. Non-pharmacologic management (i.e., enemas for constipation, use of oxygen, physical therapy, etc.)

J. Efficacy of pain management (and ability to assess and revise treatment plan, i.e., adjust therapies for desired effect).

From: Meekin SA, Klein JE, Fleischman AR, and Fins JJ. Development of a Palliative Education Assessment Tool for Medical Student Education. *Academic Medicine* 75(10)(2000):986–992.

Public Perspectives on Pain and Meaning

There is much that should inform your assessment of pain. First there is the broader cultural context. How are prevailing cultural attitudes toward pain and stoicism affecting your patient's report of discomfort or distress? Is pain accepted as part of being ill, something that cannot be remedied? Or is pain seen as being somehow redemptive from a religious perspective? This backdrop is further complicated by barriers to pain relief held by both professionals and your patients. We have already discussed the difficulty of adequate pain management that stem from regulatory and professional barriers in Chapter 8. But patients also present barriers in their report of pain.

Patients will often underreport their distress because they want to maintain control over their symptoms. A study of outpatient attitudes towards pain provides a window on the attitudes towards palliation and pain relief that we harbor before we are confronted by life-altering illness.[64] Americans frequently experience pain and are often stoic in their response to it.[65] While most study respondents acknowledged the presence of pain in their everyday lives, they generally did not act upon it. Fully two thirds of respondents withstood "fairly serious pain" while only 30 percent "acted quickly to relieve it." In addition, subjects reported that they will engage in self-medication to avoid seeking medical care.

Both stoicism and self-care are important issues to bear in mind when talking with your patients because they point to denial and the patient's need to maintain control and avoid the spectre of serious illness. It is reassuring if one can withstand the pain without medication or if the pain can be relieved with over-the-counter drugs and without a doctor's visit. Something handled in this way is easy to dismiss as not being serious. And that is the point about the *symbolic meaning of pain*. What does this pain herald? What does it represent? Put another way, fully 88 percent of respondents reported that it was more important to treat the *cause* of the pain than the pain itself. This suggests that many are concerned more about the implications of the pain than the burden it may impose.

Patients avoid highly effective medications like morphine because of what that medication *represents*. They link its receipt to an ominous prognosis. "Morphine, isn't that what you give to *dying* patients?" This association, along with unfounded fears about becoming addicted to painkillers, can be a barrier to effective pain management and patient compliance.

Biological Symptom Assessment

Excellent works have been written on pain and symptom assessment and our objective is not to retrace this scholarship here.[66-73] Instead, the task is to review overarching principles in pain management that will aid in your evaluation of the patient's symptom burden.

A critical place to begin is to ensure that your assessment of the patient's symptoms is predicated upon a scientific understanding of pathophysiology. When considering the patient's pain, you should seek to categorize the patient's distress into one of the major pain categories (neuropathic, nocioceptive, etc.) and link this descriptor to underlying pathophysiology. This will allow you to tailor your therapeutic response in much the same way that you already choose an antibiotic for a specific microorganism. Although you might use a broad-spectrum agent to treat a common pathogen, we all agree it is best to narrow the spectrum of treatment and be precise with therapeutics. The same is true for how you might respond to the patient's pain. Treatment should be precise and logical following established protocols (see below).

Similarly, when confronted with a patient with delirium or change in mental status, you need to be precise in your diagnostic assessment so that you can attempt to treat and palliate the symptom most effectively. It goes without saying that you should be careful with your evaluation. Start with the patient's physiology and engage in a review of etiologies for the patient's delirium. Is it a consequence of hypercalcemia, hypoxia, or fever? Do not *presume* that a change in mental status is because the patient is on opioid analgesia.

This is a critical point because opioids are frequently blamed for mental status changes when in fact they are not causal. A paper from MD Anderson Cancer Center highlights the tendency to ignore more common causes of altered mental status such as metabolic encephalopathy, infection, and brain metastases and to falsely assume that the etiology of the delirium is opioid overdose.[74] This leads to the inappropriate overuse of opioid antagonists like naloxone,[75] which can have dire side-effects, and a failure to correctly assess—and potentially—reverse the cause of an altered mental status.

When speaking to your patients about their pain you should identify its characteristics, frequency, intensity, and site and what prompts it to occur. Historically, when did it start? What prompted it? Are they currently comfortable at rest? Do they have incident pain that is triggered by movement or a dressing change? Is the pain chronic or is it acute? Questions about the nature and intensity of their pain will help you respond therapeutically.

It is helpful to use an *analog scale* that asks the patient to rate their pain, typically on a one to ten scale, to evaluate their level of discomfort and the efficacy of your pain management.[76] But when you do this it is important to believe what the patient tells you about the degree of their pain. Studies have shown that clinicians undervalue or discount the patient's self-report of pain by one to two points on the analog scale.[77] Remember, it is the *patient's experience and perception of pain* that should guide your therapeutic response, not how much pain you think the patient should be experiencing.

In addition, in your history and physical you will want to try and link the patient's symptoms with disease specific syndromes that may be related to the diagnosis, for example, the neuropathy seen in diabetes or AIDs or the lytic bone pain you might encounter in metastatic breast cancer. Disease related symptoms can also produce neuropsychiatric syndromes such as a delirium from hypercalcemia or AIDs related dementia.

Whatever the symptom, you will want to be familiar with its onset and time course and how it has—or has not—been evaluated. What has brought the patient relief? What sort of medication has been given? What sort of side effects has the patient experienced from the use of medications? If the patient has had pain and received morphine, did he become nauseous? Is the patient too sedated and unable to interact with the family? Is the patient constipated?

Each of these side effects has a potential remedy that may be employed if you have allowed yourself to become aware of the problem. Nausea from morphine might productively be addressed by a switch to a synthetic opioid. Excess sedation can be remedied with the use of a psychostimulant like methylphenidate hydrochloride and constipation can be handled with the appropriate use of laxatives.

Be specific in your collection of this information and obtain current doses of medications and route of delivery (by mouth, IV, or topical patch, in the case of opioids) so that you will know how to appropriately escalate therapy when adding or switching opioids to decrease side-effects.

In this escalation you will want to use opioids as suggested by the WHO.[78] The opioid "ladder" is a sequence for analgesia dosing. Pain categories and appropriate therapies are broken down into three categories. For mild to moderate pain, non-opioid analgesia like acetaminophen or a nonsteroidal anti-inflammatory agent is recommended possibly along with an adjuvant therapy such as a tri-cyclic antidepressant or an anxiolytic, depending upon circumstances. For moderate pain, a weak opioid is recommended along with adjuvant therapy as needed. Stronger opioids are recommended for more severe pain.

In addition, you will want to increase your dose of opioid with adequate increments. It is important to recall several basic issues when considering dosing. The first is the issue of *prn* versus around the clock dosing. For chronic pain at the end of life, it is far better to provide around the clock dosing with a basal amount of opioid to avoid the peaks and troughs that can occur with *prn* dosing. Twenty-four hour dosing avoids recurrence of pain during troughs and the possibility of withdrawal because levels are sustained. Basal levels of opioid can be augmented with prn doses for unexpected pain or as a pre-medication prior to a procedure. Short-acting, immediate release preparations of opioids can be used for this purpose.

The second issue related to dosing is the amount of medication. It is important to appreciate that patients will become tolerant to their dose of opioid and require escalating doses. Even if their pain burden was in a steady state and not progressing, patients will need increasing doses of opioids simply because they are becoming more tolerant of their present dose. Second, patients at the end of life who experience pain see an escalation of their distress. This increase in pain generally reflects the progression of their disease, for example their tumor burden.

These two factors—tolerance and disease progression— will necessitate increases in dosing that you may believe to be excessive, dangerous, or even illegal, because you feel that you are hastening death. Despite your feelings, using appropriate increases in opioid analgesia is good medical practice and a professional obligation. They are not excessive because of increasing tolerance. While a large dose of opioid analgesia would be dangerous in a patient who is opioid naive, chronically dosed patients develop increasing tolerance thus muting the drug's efficacy and physiologic effects. There is no categorical safe dose of morphine. It all depends upon the patient, the history, and symptom burden.

We have already reviewed the legal issues as they relate to the use of pain medication at the end of life in Chapter 3 and refer you there should you want to pursue these questions in more detail. Suffice it to say here that the appropriate use of opioids is accepted medical practice and that some legal scholars have inferred a constitutional right to palliative care—including pain relief—in Supreme Court rulings on assisted suicide.[79]

Finally, determine whether the patient has received any non-pharmacological modalities to pain such as radiation or physical therapy or employed complementary and alternative medicine approaches such as acupuncture.[80,81] It is estimated that a large percentage of patients near the end of life utilize complementary and alternative medicine interventions.[82] Because of potential interactions between medications and supplements, you need to be certain to collect this history.[83] It is critical to avoid becoming judgmental about complementary and alternative medicine approaches even if you do not endorse their use so that you are able to collect this information.[84]

If your patient feels that you will judge them harshly because they have sought treatments outside of the conventional Western paradigm, they may withhold the information, and you might not learn what you need in order to provide proper care. You might not appreciate potential drug–supplement interactions or understand why they have sought out alternative "healers" and are desperate for the cure, for salvation. Seen this way, the use of complementary and alternative medicine might be taken as a symptom of a deeper set of issues that will call upon you and your skills.

References

1 Fins JJ, Guest RS, and Acres CA. Gaining Insight into the Care of Hospitalized Dying Patients: An Interpretative Narrative Analysis. *Journal of Pain and Symptom Management* 20(6)(2000):399–407.

2 Solomon MZ. How Physicians Talk About Futility: Making Words Mean Too Many Things. *The Journal of Law, Medicine & Ethics* 21(2) (1993):231–237.

3 Sulmasy DP, Dwyer M, Marx E. Do the Ward Notes Reflect the Quality of End-of-Life Care? *Journal of Medical Ethics* 22(6)(1996):344–348.

4 Stead Jr., EA, Wagner GS, Cebe B, and Rozear MP, eds. *E.A. Stead, Jr. What This Patient Needs is a Doctor.* Durham: Carolina Academic Press, 1978: 29.

5 Fins JJ. Advance Directives and SUPPORT. *Journal of the American Geriatrics Society* 45(4)(1997):519–520.

6 Fins JJ. When the Prognosis Leads to Indifference. *Journal of Palliative Medicine* 5(4)(2002):571–573.

7 Scott PA. Autonomy, Power and Control in Palliative Care. *Cambridge Quarterly of Healthcare Ethics* 8(2)(1999):139–147.

8 Christakis NA. *Death Foretold: Prophecy and Prognosis in Medical Care.* Chicago: The University of Chicago Press, 1999: 41.

9 Solomon MZ, O'Donnell L, Jennings B, et al. Decisions Near the End of Life: Professional Views on Life-Sustaining Treatments. *American Journal of Public Health* 83(1)(1993):14–23.

10 Fins JJ and Nilson EG. An Approach to Educating Residents about Palliative Care and Clinical Ethics. *Academic Medicine* 75(6)(2000): 662–665.

11 Cowan P. In the Land of the Sick. *The Village Voice.* May 17, 1988.

12 Thayer WS. Osler, the Teacher. In *Sir William Osler, Bart.: Brief Tributes to his Personality, Influence and Public Service.* Baltimore: Johns Hopkins University Press, 1920: 51–54. As cited in JA Barondess. Is Osler Dead? *Perspectives in Biology and Medicine* 45(1)(2002):65–84.

13 Christakis NA and Iwashyna TJ. Attitude and Self-reported Practice Regarding Prognostication in a National Sample of Internists. *Archives of Internal Medicine* 158(21)(1998):2389–2395.

14 Drought TS. Presentation to Division of Medical Ethics, Weill Medical College of Cornell University, May 7, 2004.

15 Kuhl D. *What Dying People Want: Practical Wisdom for the End of Life.* New York: Public Affairs, 2002: 241–242.

16 Lunney JR, Lynn J, Foley DJ. Patterns of Functional Decline at the End of Life. *Journal of the American Medical Association* 289(19)(2003): 2387–2392.

17 Fins JJ, Miller FG, Acres CA, et al. End-of-Life Decision-Making in the Hospital: Current Practices and Future Prospects. *Journal of Pain and Symptom Management* 17(1)(1999):6–15.

18 Case description based on a presentation by Dr. Russell Portenoy at the New York State Judicial Institute, June 9, 2004.

19 Katz M, Abbey S, Rydall A, et al. Psychiatric Consultation for Competency to Refuse Medical Treatment: A Retrospective Study of Patient Characteristics and Outcome. *Psychosomatics* 36(1)(1995):33–41.

20 Lawlor PG, Fainsinger RL, and Bruera ED. Delirium at the End of Life: Critical Issues in Clinical Practice and Research. *Journal of the American Medical Association* 15(19)(2000):2427–2429.

21 Sullivan MD and Youngner SJ. Depression, Competence and the Right to Refuse Lifesaving Medical Treatment. *American Journal of Psychiatry* 151(7)(1994):971–978.

22 Zaubler TS, Viederman M, and Fins JJ. Ethical, Legal, and Psychiatric Issues in Capacity, Competence, and Informed Consent: An Annotated Bibliography of Representative Articles. *General Hospital Psychiatry* 18(3)(1996):155–172.

23 Toombs SK. *The Meaning of Illness: A Phenomenological Account of the Different Perspectives of Physician and Patient.* Boston: Kluwer Academic Publishers, 1992:26–27.

24 Shakespeare W. *Hamlet.* Act II, Scene I, lines 66–71. *The Norton Shakespeare.* Greenblatt S, Cohen W, Howard JE, and Eisaman Maus K, (Eds.) New York: W.W. Norton & Company, 1997:1705.

25 Wood S. (Director). *Pride of the Yankees.* HBO Studios. ASIN 6303597874. Video Release Date: September 23, 1997. Original Release date, 1943.

26 Rosenbaum JR, Bradley EH, Holboe ES, et al. Sources of Ethical Conflict in Medical Housestaff Training: A Qualitative Study. *American Journal of Medicine* 116(6)(2004):402–407.

27 Fallowfield LJ, Jenkins VA, and Beveridge HA. Truth May Hurt but Deceit Hurts More: Communication in Palliative Care. *Palliative Medicine* 16(4)(2002):297–303.

28 Buckman R. *How to Break Bad News.* Baltimore: The Johns Hopkins University Press, 1992.

29 Buckman R. Communication Skills in Palliative Care: A Practical Guide. *Neurologic Clinics* 19(4)(2001):989–1004.

30 Barondess JA. Is Osler Dead? *Perspectives in Biology and Medicine* 45(1)(2002):65–84.

31 Blackhall LJ, Murphy ST, Frank G, et al. Ethnicity and Attitudes toward Patient Autonomy. *Journal of the American Medical Association* 274(10)(1995):820–825.

32 Blackhall LJ, Frank G, Murphy ST, et al. Ethnicity and Attitudes towards Life Sustaining Technology. *Social Science & Medicine* 48(12)(1999):1779–1789.

33 The SUPPORT Principal Investigators. A Controlled Trial to Improve Care for Seriously Ill Hospitalized Patients. *Journal of the American Medical Association* 274(20)(1995):1591–1598.

34 Fins JJ, Peres J, Schumacher JD and Meier C. *On the Road from Theory to Practice: Progressing Towards Seamless Palliative Care.* Washington, DC: Last Acts National Program Office, Robert Wood Johnson Foundation, 2003.

35 DNR Orders: Honoring Do Not Resuscitate Orders. South Jersey Ethics Alliance, the New Jersey Department of Health, and MICU (Mobile Intensive Care Units). *New Jersey Medicine* 93(3)(1997):140–144.

36 Jaslow D, Barbera JA, Johnson E, et al. Termination of Nontraumatic Cardiac Arrest Resuscitative Efforts in the Field: A National Survey. *Academic Emergency Medicine* 4(9)(1997):904–907.

37 Clemency MV and Thompson NJ. 'Do Not Resuscitate' (DNR) Orders and the Anesthesiologist: A Survey. *Anesthesia and Analgesia* 76(2)(1993):394–401.

38 Troug RD. 'Do-Not-Resuscitate Orders' during Anesthesia and Surgery. *Anesthesiology* 74(3)(1991):606–608.

39 Olsson GL and Hall B. Cardiac Arrest during Anaethesia. *Acta Anaesthesiologica Scandinavia* 32(8)(1988):653–664.

40 Peatfield RC, Sillett RW, Taylor D, et al. Survival after Cardiac Arrest in Hospital. *Lancet* 1(8024)(1977):1223–1225.

41 State of New York. DOH Memorandum 11/2/92. *Health Facilities Series*: H-27; RHCF-22; HHA-19; Hospice 10.

42 Cohen CB & Cohen P. Do-Not-Resuscitate Orders in the Operating Room. *New England Journal of Medicine* 325(26)(1991):1879–1882.

43 Statement of the American College of Surgeons on Advance Directives by Patients: 'Do Not Resuscitate' in the OR. *ACS Bulletin*, September 1994:29.

44 Lindemann Nelson J. Families and Futility. *Journal of the American Geriatrics Society* 42(8)(1994):879–882.

45 Fins JJ. Futility in Clinical Practice: Report on a Congress of Clinical Societies. *Journal of the American Geriatrics Society* 42(8)(1994): 861–865

46 Thompson BL, Lawson D, Croughan-Minihane M, et al. Do Patients' Ethnic and Social Factors Influence the Use of Do-Not-Resuscitate Orders? *Ethnicity of Disease* 9(1)(1999):132–139.

47 Shepardson LB, Gordon HS, Ibrahim SA, et al. Racial Variation in the Use of Do-not-resuscitate Orders. *Journal of General Internal Medicine* 14(1)(1999):15–20.

48 Hornberger JC, Gibson CD, Wood W, et al. Eliminating Language Barriers for Non-English-speaking Patients. *Medical Care* 34(8)(1996): 845–856.

49 Haffner L. Translation Is not Enough: Interpeting in a Medical Setting. *Western Journal of Medicine* 157(3)(1992):255–259.

50 I am indebted to a segment on the National Public Radio's show, *The Infinite Mind*, which addressed cross cultural and translation issues in psychiatry for insights into this topic. Show aired on WNYC-FM on April 17, 2004.

51 This section is excerpted and based upon: Fins JJ. Approximation and Negotiation: Clinical Pragmatism and Difference. *Cambridge Quarterly of Healthcare Ethics* 7(1)(1998):68–76.

52 New York State Department of Health. *Determination of Death.* Adopted Regulation 10 N.Y.C.R.R. 400.16.

53 The New Jersey Declaration of Death Act. P.L. 1991, Chapter 90. (To be codified as Chapter 6A of Title 26 of the Revised Statutes.) Section 5(1998): Exemption to Accomodate Personal Religious Beliefs. *Kennedy Institute of Ethics Journal* 1(4)(1991):289–292.

54 Uniform Determination of Death Act. 12 *Uniform Laws Annotated 320* (1990 Supp.).

55 Fins JJ. Breaking the Silence: Futility, Fear and Anger. In *Futility, Decisions Near the End of Life*, vol. 7. Solomon MZ, Jennings BJ, Crigger BJ, et al., (Eds.) Newton, MA: Education Development Center, Inc. 1997.

56 Ad Hoc Committee of the Harvard Medical School to Examine the Definition of Brain Death. A Definition of Irreversible Coma. *Journal of the American Medical Association* 205(6)(1968):337–340.

57 Veatch RM. The Impending Collapse of the Whole-Brain Definition of Death. *Hastings Center Report* 23(4)(1993):18–24.

58 Troug RD and Fackler JC. Rethinking Brain Death. *Critical Care Medicine* 20(12)(1992):1705–1713.

59 Brenner D, Blanchard T, Fins JJ and Hirschfield B. *Embracing Life and Facing Death: A Jewish Guide to Palliative Care.* New York: CLAL—The National Jewish Center for Learning and Leadership, 2002.

60 Rosner F. Definition of Death. *Modern Medicine and Jewish Ethics: Second Revised and Augmented Edition.* New York: Yeshiva University Press, 1991:263–275.

61 Fins JJ. Across the Divide: Religious Objections to Brain Death. *Journal of Religion and Health* 34(1)(1995):33–39.

62 Meekin SA, Klein JE, Fleischman AR, et al. Development of a Palliative Education Assessment Tool for Medical Student Education. *Academic Medicine* 75(10)(2000):986–992.

63 Wood EB, Meekin SA, Fins JJ, et al. Enhancing Palliative Care Education in Medical School Curricula: Implementation of the Palliative Education Assessment Tool. *Academic Medicine* 77(4)(2002):285–291.

64 Bostrom M. Summary of Mayday Fund Survey: Public Attitudes about Pain and Analgesics. *Journal of Pain and Symptom Management* 13(3)(1997):166–168.

65 Fins JJ. Public Attitudes about Pain and Analgesics: Clinical Implications. *Journal of Pain and Symptom Management* 13(3)(1997):169–171.

66 Foley KM. Pain Assessment and Cancer Pain Syndromes. *Oxford Textbook of Palliative Medicine*, 2nd Edition. Doyle D, Hanks GWC, and MacDonald N, Eds. New York: Oxford University Press, 1998:310–331.

67 Payne R, Pharmacologic Management of Pain. In *Principles and Practice of Supportive Oncology*, Berger AM, Portenoy RK, Weissman DE, (Eds.) Philadelphia, PA: Lippincott Williams & Wilkins, 1998.

68 Hanks G and Cherny N. Opioid Analgesic Therapy. *Oxford Textbook of Palliative Medicine*, 2nd edition. Doyle D, Hanks GWC, and MacDonald N, (Eds.) New York: Oxford University Press, 1998:331–355.

69 Max MB and Payne R (Cmte chairs). *Principles of Analgesic Use in the Treatment of Acute Pain and Cancer Pain.* 4th ed., American Pain Society, Lakeview, IL, 1999.

70 Potenoy RK. *Contemporary Diagnosis and Management of Pain in Oncologic and AIDS Patients.* Newton, PA: Handbooks in Health Care Co., 1997.

71 Doyle D, Hanks G, Cherry NI, and Calman K, (Eds.) *Oxford Textbook of Palliative Medicine*, 3rd edition. New York: Oxford University Press, 2005.

72 Ballantyne JC, Fishman SM, and Abdi S, (Eds.) *The Massachusetts General Hospital Handbook of Pain Management*, 2nd ed. Philadelphia: Lippincott Williams & Wilkins, 2002.

73 Abrahm JL. *A Physician's Guide to Pain and Symptom Management in Cancer Patients.* Baltimore: Johns Hopkins University Press, 2002.

74 Manfredi PL, Ribeiro S, Chandler SW, et al. Inappropriate Use of Naloxone in Cancer Pain. *Journal of Pain and Symptom Management* 11(2)(1996):131–134.

75 Fins JJ. Acts of Omission and Commission in Pain Management: The Ethics of Naloxone Use. *Journal of Pain and Symptom Management* 17(2)(1999):120–124.

76 Fishman B, Pasternak S, Wallenstein SL, et al. The Memorial Pain Assessment Card. A Valid Instrument for the Evaluation of Cancer Pain. *Cancer* 60(5)(1987):1151–1158.

77 Drayer RA, Henderson J and Reidenberg M. Barriers to Better Pain Control in Hospitalized Patients. *Journal of Pain and Symptom Management* 17(6)(1999):434–440.

78 World Health Organization. *Cancer Pain Relief with a Guide to Opioid Availability*, 2nd Edition. Geneva: WHO, 1996.

79 Burt RA. The Supreme Court speaks—Not Assisted Suicide but a Constitutional Right to Palliative Care. *New England Journal of Medicine* 337(17)(1997):1234–1236.

80 Konski A, Feigenberg S, and Chow E. Palliative Radiation Therapy. *Seminars in Oncology* 32(2)(2005):156–164.

81 Cheville AL. Cancer Rehabilitation. *Seminars in Oncology* 32(2)(2005): 219–224.

82 Pan CX, Morrison RS, Ness J, et al. Complementary and Alternative Medicine in the Management of Pain, Dyspnea, and Nausea and Vomiting Near the End of Life. A Systematic Review. *Journal of Pain and Symptom Management* 20(5)(2000):374–387.

83 Tilden VP, Drach LL, and Tolle SW. Complementary and Alternative Therapy Use at the End-of-Life in Community Settings. *Journal of Alternative and Complementary Medicine* 10(5)(2004):811–817.

84 *White House Commission on Complementary and Alternative Medicine Policy, Final Report.* Washington, DC: U.S. Government Printing Office, 2002.

c h a p t e r   t e n

Formulating the Goals of Care

Introduction

It should be obvious by now that the formulation of goals of care requires deep knowledge of the clinical and narrative details of the case. They may not be obvious ahead of time but emerge through hard work and careful reflection. The goals should emerge after collecting this information just as a conventional clinical diagnosis is made after a detailed history, physical exam, and formulation of the differential diagnosis. And as the diagnosis determines the plan for care, so too, the goals determine the treatment plan. *Goals should drive the therapy—therapy should not drive the goals.*

GOALS OF CARE:

Cure   [ ]

Restore Function   [ ]

Prolong Life   [ ]

Comfort Care/Palliation   [ ]

Comments: _____

Figure 10.1

Defining Goals

Goals, simply put, are objectives that you are helping your patient meet over the course of an illness. They can take a number of shapes and can evolve over time as the patient's course of disease evolves. Because goals can change, it is important to link these objectives to the patient's prognosis (see Chapter 8). Differing stages may call for permutations in these goals. At the outset, the clear objective will likely be the pursuit of cure. Towards the end of life, comfort and palliation may predominate, although some patients and families will never want to cede to illness and want to press on with care geared towards cure. There may also be situations where some clinicians believe that further aggressive interventions may offer the chance of a cure, or add years to the patient's life, though the patient and family may view continued treatment too burdensome in the face of a low likelihood of success.

Whatever the particular dynamics informing the care of the individual patient, the art of patient care is to try and help patients and families *realize their unique goals*. This is easier said than done because in most health care encounters a discussion of goals never occurs. They are taken for granted and are implicit. Early in life, the goal may be prevention through childhood vaccination. Later in adulthood, it might be the pursuit of a cure for cancer or the repair of an injured meniscus.

In each of these cases, the unspoken objective is the maintenance of health, which is taken as the norm. In childhood, the goal is to avoid death from a preventable illness. Clearly childhood death would constitute a deviation from what is expected and what, in the modern era, has become the norm. As an adult, it is to *return* to the norm of health by arthroscoping a knee or excising a tumor as indicated by the etymology of "cure," which means to take care of, to cleanse, or rid of an infirmity.[1]

Because cure or the closely related functional notion of restoring the patient to their premorbid function are the unspoken goals of care for most encounters with physicians and the health care system, it is rare for patients and their families to suggest that comfort measures and palliative care are to be pursued. Unless they have witnessed care for a loved one who died comforted by hospice care or a palliative care program, they have not been acculturated to think about palliative care as a goal of care.

Your task is to help patients and families gradually make the transition from the unspoken—and often unexamined—notions of care that have motivated their encounters with medicine to a consideration of the merits of palliative care. Goals are not revisited in the face of terminal illness; patients continue to receive aggressive curative measures that inflict significant burden though they have little chance of succeeding. Socrates once reflected that "the unexamined life is not worth living." Invoking this sentiment, life in an ICU with an intractable solid tumor, septic and unconscious on a ventilator may be an unexamined life that emerges as one that is no longer not worth living after further reflection.

In a compassionate and kind way, you should help patients avoid this common, and I would add, often tragic scenario. With compassion and *knowledge from the goal-setting process* help patient and family assess their goals and consider the merits of palliative care, *from their perspective*. Your approach should not be to proselytize, but to help patient and family see how adoption of a palliative approach might help them achieve what remain as achievable goals.

A helpful way to frame your discussions of palliative goals of care is to return to the World Health Organization (WHO) definition of palliative care that we first considered in Chapter 2. After speaking of pain and symptom management in the face of disease which is not responsive to cure, the definition concludes with the simple objective that "The goal of palliative care is the achievement of the best quality of life for patients and their families."[2]

The WHO articulation of the goal of palliation is a useful over-arching heuristic because it suggests that curative, rehabilitative, or palliative approaches to care may be employed individually or in tandem to help achieve the best quality of life for patient and family. This is an important and often overlooked point. Although we often speak of a palliative approach to care, in reality, most of the time we are pursuing a mosaic or blended approach to care utilizing the best available interventions to make the patient comfortable. Strategies sometimes employed to achieve cure, such as radiation therapy, are used alongside comfort measures such as opioid analgesia to promote comfort care goals. So too can surgical and rehabilitative strategies be used to improve the functional status of a patient with a terminal illness. Consider the patient who undergoes orthopedic surgery to pin a pathological hip fracture from metastatic disease who receives physical therapy to improve mobility, functional status, and quality of life.

A mosaic approach to care is also helpful because it will allow you to titrate the mix of palliative to curative. If we return to the graphic on futility that we first encountered in Chapter 4 (reproduced below), we will recall how these disputes evolve when there are discordant expectations about the goals of care.

Viewing the emergence of palliation into a disease trajectory as a sort of titration is helpful because it allows patient

Figure 10.2
From, Fins JJ. Principles in Palliative Care: An Overview.
Journal of Respiratory Care 2000; 45(11): 1320–1330.

LESSONS FROM FUTILITY DISPUTES

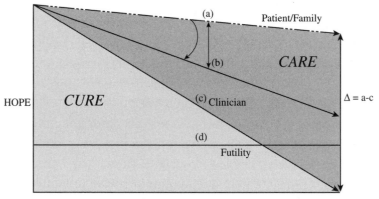

and family to adjust gradually to a changing balance of "curing" and "caring." The concentration of curative strategies is diluted by a palliative approach to care so that over time, palliation predominates.

A gradual transition from the curative to the palliative is critically important *because palliative care is never anyone's first choice as a care strategy*. It best becomes a viable alternative over time, incrementally and in small doses. One way to help patients and families make this transition is to help them articulate *intermediate goals of care*.

One such goal is the prolongation of life in the absence of a definitive curative therapy. This goal takes into account that cure is no longer possible but that temporizing therapies remain that can allow the patient to live longer, perhaps with a lesser sense of well-being. This will be the case with many chronic or degenerative diseases, such as advanced heart failure or a slowly progressive chronic leukemia. Though the patient may require diuretics or periodic transfusion to remain comfortable, life remains tolerable.

Alternately, life can be prolonged for days or weeks with aggressive life-sustaining therapies when death is more imminent. In both of these situations it is important to be clear in the goals of care, lest the patient or family mistake temporizing measures as being curative. Again, a failure to distinguish therapies employed from goals pursued, can lead to misconstruals and disputes over medical futility as was noted in Chapter 4 and illustrated in Figure 4.1.

Once comfort care or palliation becomes the predominant or single goal, this orientation can provide a framework for care decisions. Guided by a clarity about goals, interventions that promote pain and symptom management can be continued and those that do not can be stopped. At one end of the spectrum, this may call for the escalation of opioid analgesia to promote pain relief. At the other, it may lead to a decision to remove life-sustaining therapy.

Having clear goals of care can be extremely helpful in making sure that the care plan is internally consistent, an issue that can become especially important when decisions to withdraw care are made. Consider the case of an elderly man with gastric carcinoma. He was admitted two weeks earlier after he collapsed at home. By the time he arrived in the Emergency Room he was pulseless. He was resuscitated and subsequent evaluation revealed coffee ground emesis, melanotic stool, and a profound anemia. The patient was transferred to the MICU and underwent an emergency endoscopy to identify the course of bleeding and was found to have a large gastric carcinoma. Bleeding was controlled but his subsequent course was marked by multi-system organ failure including adult respiratory distress syndrome, acute renal failure, as well as anoxic encephalopathy. The patient received hemodynamic and ventilatory support and underwent two sessions of hemodialysis.

After one week of ICU care, the intensivist initiated a discussion with the patient's wife to consider a DNR order and to initiate "comfort care measures." The plan was to withhold dialysis and transfer him out of the unit but *maintain mechanical ventilation*. The intensivist had limited the discussion to the withdrawal of dialysis and did not broach the issue of the ventilator, in part, because he did not want the patient to die immediately in his unit.

The patient's wife did not know enough to question this care plan and believed that the decision to stop dialysis was going to be sufficient to lead to the end of the patient's suffering. She fully expected that death was going to be imminent with transfer out of the unit and with the halting of dialysis.

She asked for the assistance of the ethics consultation service because the patient remained alive a week after transfer out of the ICU. She reported that she told the inten-sivist that she wanted to abide by her husband's wishes and keep him comfortable if there was no hope for recovery. She is distraught that he is still alive and suffering. She reports having been told by the intensivist that the patient would expire "two to three days after all the tubes had come out."

Tragically, for the patient and his wife, "all the tubes" did not come out. The care plan was internally inconsistent with a decision to maintain one life-sustaining therapy (the venti-lator) and not the other (dialysis). Here, a failure to fully agree on the goals of care, led to the all too common scenario of the therapies driving the goals and not the goals of care directing the use of available therapies. Unfortunately, in this case, the intensivist was uncomfortable with the decision to withdraw the ventilator though he was comfortable stopping the dialysis.

A more deliberate articulation of the goals of care would have helped to make it clear that it was ethically consistent—and appropriate—to withdraw the ventilator, given the gravity of the situation and the patient's previously expressed preferences. Indeed it would have also illustrated that both extubation and the cessation of dialysis were with-drawals of life-sustaining therapy in a patient who was venti-latory dependent and anuric and going to die of renal failure. Finally, it would have allowed the staff to support the family in the patient's final days and ameliorate the sense of aban-donment that the wife sensed after the husband was trans-ferred from the ICU to the step-down unit.

Hospital Resources

Once the goals of care have been articulated, they need to be implemented just as a therapeutic response follows from a diagnosis. In the hospital setting, responding therapeutically often means calling upon other professionals to provide additional assistance with patient care. Alternately, if you have been unable to adequately define the goals of care, there are other professionals in the hospital who can be of help, both diagnostically and therapeutically.

In this section we will briefly review the services that your colleagues may be able to provide and suggest strategies that you can employ to optimize these referrals. Each of these areas of sub-specialty care are deserving of a book-length discussion. Our purpose here is to suggest how their involvement in the care of your patients can be of assistance and how and when you should ask for their help, not to provide a comprehensive review of these disciplines.

Planned Interventions	Comments:
Psychiatry Consult [ ]	_____
Pastoral Care Visit [ ]	_____
Pain Service/Palliative Care Consult [ ]	_____
Referral to Palliative Care Unit [ ]	_____
Hospice Referral [ ]	_____
Social Work [ ]	_____
Ethics Committee [ ]	_____
Other [ ]	_____

Figure 10.3

Psychiatry Consultation

Psychiatrists who consult on medical and surgical patients in the general hospital often play an important role in end-of-life care.[3] Their service is often referred to as consultation–

liaison psychiatry, to convey their task of bringing psychiatric expertise to the care of the medically ill inpatients. One veteran practitioner has defined his field as, "the application of the usual domain of psychiatry, namely a person's feelings, thinking, and behavior to the treatment of some medical condition by another physician. The psychiatrist is the liaison between the patient and his primary treaters and any psychiatric treatment is done within that context."[4] Many of these psychiatrists have training in internal medicine as well as psychiatry and are comfortable outside the psychiatric setting.

These psychiatrists can assist with assessment of decision-making capacity and consent to treatment[5] (See Chapter 6) and help in the evaluation of patients who want to refuse life-sustaining therapies (See Chapter 9).[6-8] Because of their expertise, consultation–liaison psychiatrists can serve as arbiters of whether patients do or do not have the capacity to make medical decisions when it is clinically unclear or when there is disagreement among the medical team members.[9] These evaluations are essential to the work of hospital ethics committees, which will be discussed shortly. Indeed, sometimes clinicians confuse the role of the psychiatry consultant and that of the ethics committee. This indicates the level of interaction between these two services.[10]

Beyond these assessments of capacity, consultation–liaison psychiatry can also assist in distinguishing normal grief from clinical depression, which in terminally-ill patients is characterized by a sense of guilt, worthlessness, helplessness, hopelessness, and persistent suicidal ideation. These symptoms are more reliable indicators of depression in this population than the usual neurovegetative symptoms of depression such as anorexia, weight loss, and inability to sleep seen in a medically-well population.[11] Psychiatric consultation can also assist in the management of anxiety, delirium, and other neuropsychiatric disorders[12,13] as well as the medical management of the psychiatrically ill patient.[14]

Perhaps most critically, psychiatrists, and their colleagues in psychology, can bring their psychodynamic skills to the bedside of patients with existential questions triggered by the imminence of death.[15,16] The transition from wellness to medical illness requires patients to adapt to a new reality and may trigger maladaptive[17] or complex emotional responses such as denial, panic, and what has been described as "regressive dependency."[18] This has been defined as the scenario where the formerly independent adult now finds himself dependent upon others for care and comfort. Some patients will not allow themselves to fall into dependent roles and this can lead to noncompliance that may complicate care and lead to depression. Psychiatrists can help patients cope with their altered circumstances by helping to place their current illnesses into the context of their psychodynamic life narratives.[19] This narrative contextualization

> is designed to create a new perspective and to increase self-esteem through the emphasis of past strengths, support of coping mechanisms that have been effective in the past; and where applicable, it is designed to point out that the depression is an understandable response when previous adaptive methods can no longer be used.[20]

These interventions can be therapeutic by helping patients find meaning in their remaining days. You can be of tremendous help to your patients, and their families, by identifying the psychiatric and psychological dimensions of their illness and seeking appropriate consultations with psychiatry when it is needed.

Pastoral Care/Chaplaincy

Surveys have indicated that patients near the end of life frequently seek counsel and comfort from their religious faith.[21] Even those who have led a secular existence often turn to their religious heritage at life's end.[22]

To meet the spiritual needs of patients and families, the Joint Commission on Accreditation of Healthcare Organizations (JCAHO) that accredits hospitals requires that hospitals make pastoral care or chaplaincy services available to their patients.[23] The benefit and importance of pastoral care may be unappreciated, and their services may be underutilized. You may feel intimidated by clergy in the hospital setting and be uncomfortable working with them.[24] You should put these reservations aside and get to know the chaplain in your hospital or on your clinical service and readily offer your patients the opportunity to meet with them.

Chaplaincy services can help you do a better job of helping patient and family, especially when you are caring for those who are from different religious traditions. Their services become increasingly important, as the hospital has become the gathering place for our modern society. Perhaps nowhere else do people of such different backgrounds and faith traditions come together equally humbled and transformed by illness and infirmity. This rich convocation of diverse peoples, cultures, and religious traditions has made our collective deliberations about life and death more complicated and nuanced.

Hospital chaplains can come from the community or be graduates of pastoral care residencies. Some will even be boarded by the College of Chaplains. Although chaplains from local churches, synagogues, or mosques can bring expertise and comfort to inpatients, hospital based chaplains have the added advantage of having their fulltime ministry in the clinical setting. They come to understand the medical context and the culture of care experienced by patients. Over time they gain the trust of physicians and nurses and can help serve as an intermediary between the patient and family and the clinical team. They can also identify patients who might need the additional expertise of a psychiatrist.

Many hospital-based chaplains are as skilled in counseling as they are informed about theology and are thus able to provide psychological as well as spiritual support to patients and families. Pastoral care services are generally multi-faith. Theirs is an ecumenical ministry, an embrace of diversity, that is especially well-suited to the increasing number of blended families that will congregate around the bedside.

You will find that hospital-based chaplains will tend to be less doctrinaire about decisions at the end of life because they have spent more time at the bedside ministering to the dying and seek to find common ground and common cause with their medical colleagues.[25]

In my experience, hospital-based chaplains will tend to put patient comfort first and not embrace, for example, a theological stance that maintains that untreated pain is somehow redemptive. This perspective seeks to relate the suffering of the patient to the sacrifice of Christ on the cross. Although the view is that self-abnegation will hasten salvation, from a clinical perspective, the forgoing of pain medication is exceedingly corrosive to patient care. I view it as a violation of a basic human right to be free of treatable pain. To willingly deprive a patient of pain relief strikes me as a violation of the physician's obligation to promote beneficence and patient well-being.

From a practical standpoint, the withholding of pain relief will cause patients to suffer needlessly, making it difficult for them to attend to prayer and spiritual issues. From a theological perspective, it is a stance that is also suspect and countered by verse from the Gospels that can be interpreted to mean that patients who are in pain should be treated. From the Book of Matthew, "Those who are well do not need a physician, but the sick do" (Matthew, 9:12) and "Go and learn the meaning of the words, 'I desire mercy, not sacrifice.' I did not come to call the righteous but sinners." (Matthew, 9:13). And from the physician, Luke, "For everyone who asks, receives: and the one who seeks, finds; and to the one who knocks, the door will be opened." (Luke, 11:10)[26] James Drane, a former priest and author of a volume advancing a liberal Catholic bioethics, has written eloquently about the moral obligation to treat pain.

> There is no cure for dying; but the best, the safest, the most certainly effective palliative care is provided by physical relief and by staying with dying patients in a perceptive and compassionate way . . . Protection against suffering from despair at the end of life comes from being able to look beyond death. To be able to look beyond death with faith and hope toward a future is most likely in the presence of caring and compassionate others.[27]

This is a stance also taken by the Catholic Health Association in its writings on palliative care,[28] suggesting that the view that the endurance of pain is somehow redemptive is an idiosyncratic one at best.

Some patients will ask you to pray with them.[29] This request poses a number of ethical challenges. First among them is the issue of professional boundaries between doctor and patient.[30] Whether or not each is of the same, or differing religious tradition, joint prayer can change the usual dyadic relationship between patient and doctor. Current recommendations suggest that physicians "listen respectfully" to patients and families as they articulate their religious and spiritual beliefs and attempt to appreciate how these views inform decisions about medical care. In doing so, it is important that the physician does not attempt to fulfill the role of clergy in providing religious solace or attempt to proselytize in any way.[31] Although such guidelines are open to interpretation, with some sanctioning prayer in exceptional circumstances[32] or when there is a congruence of belief systems,[33] there is a clear consensus on the role of chaplains praying with patients and their loved ones. You can demonstrate your concern for the patient's spiritual well-being by becoming familiar with your colleagues in pastoral care and making appropriate referrals on behalf of patients and their families.

Whatever the background or experience of the chaplain ministering to your patient, it is very important to talk to him or her. The Chaplain will often have a wealth of information about the patient and family and be able to better apprehend the religious and cultural forces that inform their decisions.

Pain Service/Palliative Care Consult/ Referral to Palliative Care Unit

There are many models to provide palliative care.[34,35] Many hospitals now have dedicated pain and palliative care services and/or units designed to provide specialized end-of-life care. Because these services have only recently become part of hospital culture, there is an evolving sociology about conception and design. But whatever their configuration, these services can provide expert consultation on the technical and humanistic dimensions of end-of-life care when you need assistance.

Typically these services advise on pain management, optimizing the choice of medication in order to minimize side-effects and help diagnostically in the assessment of specific pain syndromes so that a careful diagnosis can lead to more targeted therapy. Depending upon your institutional culture, the pain and palliative care service may also help to mediate disputes about end-of-life care when the goals are in conflict. This function, however, may be played by your hospital's ethics committee.

At a general conceptual level, these programs tend to be either more medical or interventional in their overall orientation. The physician leadership of the first tend to come from non-interventional specialties such as family medicine, internal medicine (often from general medicine, geriatrics, pulmonary–critical care, or hematology–oncology), neurology, or psychiatry. A second type of service has its origins in anesthesiology. A third variation on this theme is a nurse-led program, which borrows from the primary care role played by nurses in hospice care.[36]

Neither type of service has a monopoly on technically astute and humane care, but those services that are more attuned to the broader bio-psycho-social dimensions of end-of-life care do a better job of meeting patient and family needs. Those services that are more focused on interventional strategies to relieve pain, such as the placement of indwelling catheters for the delivery of opioids or the placement of nerve blocks at the exclusion of these wider concerns may not provide comprehensive end-of-life care.

Familiarize yourself with the services provided by consultants and programs in your hospital so that your patients can receive optimal care that you feel unable to provide. In addition, knowledge of pain and palliative care programs in your institution can alert you to educational opportunities, such as elective rotations, that you might want to pursue in order to broaden your own skills in palliative medicine. A required clinical rotation in clinical ethics and palliative care at Weill Medical College of Cornell University for third and fourth year medical students has been well received and provides students with a grounding in these important disciplines.[37] You would likely benefit from similar experiences in your own institution or an elective experience elsewhere. Asking the palliative care service to consult on your patients can be an excellent introduction to the educational opportunities that might be available, either as a medical student or resident.

Hospice Referral

We have discussed hospice in Chapter 7. In this section, we will consider how patients operationally make their way from inpatient care to hospice services. The truth is that patients generally do not make this journey without the involvement of their doctors who will help them to navigate the transition from acute to hospice care.

Transfer to hospice can take several forms. Patients are discharged from hospital care to either beds in the hospital that are designated as hospice beds or sent home with community-based hospice services. The former option might be ideal when the patient is too sick for transfer or needs to be stabilized for discharge. A patient, for example, might be discharged from the hospital and transferred to inhospital hospice care if acute curative care has ceased and the remaining therapeutic issue was the stabilization of a pain regimen. Alternately, a patient might remain in the hospital receiving hospice care if they require, or request, on-going services like ventilatory support, which might be unavailable at home.

Ideally, timely goal setting would allow more patients to receive hospice care earlier in their course of treatment, thus allowing for services to be provided at home. Home hospice, which accounts for over 90 percent of hospice care, is often misunderstood by patients and families. Because hospice referral is so open to misconstrual, you need to become familiar with the wide range of services that are part of the Medicare hospice benefit. They include medications delivered to the patient's home and home care visits by highly trained and compassionate nurses committed to the hospice mission. Patients are also able to receive respite care in facility-based hospices if they or their families find this necessary. And after the patient's passing, bereavement counseling is available in the year following death. As one palliative care specialist has put it, the hospice benefit is medicine's best-kept secret.[38]

In addition, it is important to stress that the acceptance of a hospice referral does not mean that patients have to give up their primary care physician. Medical oversight of enrolled patients can be retained by the referring physician or taken on by the hospice medical director. In either scenario, the medical director is available to assist with clinical management and to provide needed palliative care expertise.

In my experience, it is preferable to maintain an ongoing relationship with the patient if you feel comfortable with providing end-of-life care. The value of your preexisting relationship with patient and family cannot be overstated.

Social Work

Although an over-arching precept of palliative care is that the object of care is not just the patient, but all those affected by the patient's illness. Social workers, by virtue of their training—and the importance they place on support systems and the role of family and friends—can help play an important role in moving beyond the doctor–patient dyad and appreciating that the broader family unit is really the object of palliative care.[39]

In practice, social workers might be consulted to initiate a psycho–social assessment on a new patient, to obtain information about personal relationships, cultural background and practices, work history, or financial status. They are important resources for information about counseling and bereavement services, discharge planning, home and hospice care, insurance coverage and financial resources. Some also conduct family meetings and provide therapeutic support to family members.

Social workers are also especially well situated to help assess and address the economic burdens imposed by a terminal illness upon the family unit. Terminal illness can lead to impoverishment through job loss, spending down of savings, and the costs of medical care and social services. These challenges are not equally distributed across society, but disproportionately burdensome for some populations, most notably African-Americans, who have higher end-of-life costs than other Americans.[40]

Social workers can help lessen these burdens by maximizing the benefits that patients and families may be eligible to receive. Because they have a more systemic approach to patient and family needs, social workers can help make a system designed for the acute care needs of patients actually work for those who have chronic and life-threatening illnesses.

Although the health care system is designed to facilitate the seamless provision of complex and costly interventions like by-pass surgery, it is not designed to provide needed palliative care services across the clinical continuum of care. Social workers can make a tremendous contribution to patient and family well-being by helping to chart the movement of patient from hospital to hospice, and home, by assisting with discharge planning, and by mobilizing existing local resources which might be needed by patient and family.

An important ingredient in this work is the assessment of what sort of assets exist in the patient's home when they are discharged. Knowledge of existing resources can help identify what needs to happen so that the patient and family's bio-psychosocial and medical needs can be met in that setting. A social worker will be especially able to assess whether there are concurrent medical problems in a family member, which might make them unable to provide ongoing care to the patient upon discharge. A failure to ask social work to help you with your patients will needlessly prolong hospital admissions and may lead to patients being discharged without adequate support and services.

Ethics Committees

Even with the best of intentions and efforts at structured goal setting, ethical dilemmas can develop in the provision of care to dying patients and their families. The complexity of hospital care, the number of practitioners involved, and the diversity of patients under care all have the potential to engender conflict over values, norms, and beliefs. Fortunately, hospital ethics committees are now widely available to help identify sources of disagreement and try to negotiate a workable compromise. They are an invaluable resource for patients and families as well as clinical staff who find themselves wondering "about the right thing to do." [41] They can also be of tremendous help to you as you seek to develop your skills in medical ethics and patient care.

You need to know how these committees function and learn how to obtain their consultative services and avail yourself of their educational outreach. Gaining these skills will promote patient welfare and deepen your appreciation of the ethical dimensions of patient care. It will also enrich your own sense of professionalism and decrease the isolation that you may feel when facing an ethical dilemma in patient care.

Most ethics case consultations in the general hospital setting center around end-of-life care issues. Many of these consults relate to decisions to withhold or withdraw life-sustaining through a Do-Not-Resuscitate (DNR) order or an advance directive such as a durable power of attorney for health care or living will.

To help you work better with your hospital ethics committee, it is important for you to understand what they do. In my view, an ethics committee does not make ethical decisions about patient care. They should not dictate choices or supersede the role traditionally held within the doctor–patient–family dynamic. Instead, ethics committees should help patients, families, and clinicians with an analysis of the choices they face so that a better decision can be made. This is done through an explicit and comprehensive process of deliberation, weighing the risks and benefits of one course or another.

Ethics committees can help you and your patients in several ways. First is through direct ethics case consultation. An ethics consult can be requested by anyone who is involved in a case, be they patient or family member or junior staff nurse or senior clinician. Anyone with moral standing in a case is, in my view, entitled to request a consult, although not all stakeholders in a case should have equal standing when it comes to the choices that are made. For example, though you might be able to request the ethics committee's involvement, your views on a particularly contentious question would have less bearing than that of the patient or family.

Ethics consults can be conducted in a number of ways, either by an individual ethics consultant or by a subcommittee of the whole of the ethics committee.[42] But whatever the mode of consultation, the goal is to gather and review the relevant facts of the case, attend to due-process concerns, and seek to reach a reasonable compromise and consensus about a decision.[43] Since their introduction into the clinical setting over twenty-five years ago, standards—and key competencies—for ethics consultations have become increasingly standardized, minimizing the likelihood of idiosyncratic consultative methods from place to place.[44,45] Central to this skillset is "advanced knowledge in moral reasoning and skill in ethical analysis" as well as the ability to engage in mediation and conflict resolution to facilitate open debate.[46–48]

Ethics committees are well-positioned to help facilitate such deliberations—and help achieve a workable consensus—precisely because of how they are constituted and structured. Accreditation expectations and ethical norms require that they be diverse bodies reflecting the lay patient population being served and the wide number of professional disciplines encountered in hospital-based medicine. This includes doctors, nurses, social workers, and chaplains, as well as patient advocates and representatives from legal affairs and administration. Most committees have lay representatives from the community. Larger committees in more academic environments also often draw upon colleagues from the humanities such as philosophy, religious studies, or cultural anthropology. This diversity can substantively improve the deliberative process and avoid a group–think dynamic necessary to achieve compromise and consensus.

The opportunity for success should not be compromised by too narrow a membership on the ethics committee because, with proper deliberation, most cases brought to the ethics committee can be resolved and a compromise reached. Most conflicts brought to the committee are viewed by clinical staff as intractable and irresolvable dilemmas that are beyond the reach of conflict resolution and not as problems that might well be solved with a little bit of patience and a careful review of the facts.[49] In my experience, having been involved in over 1,500 consults over ten years as chair of an ethics committee, I am more optimistic and have seen just the opposite. Most cases can be resolved.

In our experience, approximately 75 percent of cases are resolved after our involvement. In these cases, there was no fundamental disagreement over the facts, but a misunderstanding had emerged as the complex narrative of the case unfolded. A typical case in this category might be a conflict between surrogates, say two sisters, over what their decisionally-incapacitated father would have wanted for his care. Both children are well-intentioned and only want what is best for their Dad. One wants to continue aggressive ICU-level care; the other wants to pursue palliation. Their father did not provide direct guidance about such questions and each sister is simply going with their own moral intuition about how best to proceed. The difference between the two, though, hinges upon their understanding of their father's prognosis. The one who wants to maintain ICU care believes his condition is reversible. The other is less hopeful and thinks he should go peacefully.

From this simple, yet all too common scenario, it becomes apparent that the key to conflict resolution is to provide the family with good information about likely outcomes should ICU care continue at current levels. You could argue that this is somewhat obvious; that, of course, we provide such prognostic information to patients and their families. The reality is that these issues are not always obvious at the beginning. There are often mischaracterizations and tensions that need to be negotiated so that the real issue at the crux of the disagreement can be fleshed out.

The art of ethics consultation is in sleuthing out how differing positions about care evolved, even when all involved had beneficent intentions. In cases like this one, deconstructing how the two sisters came to their views generally reveals that they had a different sense of prognosis and likely different sources of information about their father's condition. One might have heard an encouraging word from a covering resident, while the other's opinion was formed by a more pessimistic physician. Whatever the scenario, the role of the ethicist is not to prescribe a certain course of care but rather to be sure that all involved are operating off the same set of facts and off the same page. Once the two daughters hear the same set of facts, chances are they will agree on a decision about care.

Now let us change the fact pattern just a bit and consider the next sort of case that we encounter about 10–15 percent of the time. These cases are a bit more complex. Here the two daughters know the same facts about their father's prognosis but neither knows what is the right thing to do. They do not have a disagreement between each other but rather they are uncertain about what is ethically appropriate. They could agree with each other, if they could decide what should be done. Such decisions, which could emerge over a decision to move from curative to palliative care, will remain ethically challenging, but the involvement of an ethics committee can help elucidate the facts and help ensure that all points of view were considered and that all were heard. In my experience, a complete and robust deliberative process can provide reassurance to those who are involved that the weightiness of any decision was matched by a comprehensive analysis. Although no one is entirely comfortable with the decision that was reached, all are reassured that it was a reasonable decision and a choice that was the product of a worthy process of reflection.

In a small percentage of cases, perhaps 10 percent, it becomes impossible to achieve a workable consensus. These cases can either stem from intractable family dynamics (please see the discussion of symbionic families in Chapter 9) or from a fundamental ethical disagreement amongst the parties about a contentious issue upon which society itself is unable to agree. The *Schiavo* Case, alluded to in Chapter 3, has elements of both: a divided family and a family divided over the sanctity of life and the place of patient choice. As that tragic tale illustrates, cases like that one are better to prevent than to mediate.

This breakdown in the types of cases encountered by an ethics committee illustrates that upwards of 85–90 percent can be resolved with a careful review and explication of the facts as well as efforts at mediation. This illustrates the original point that most ethics "dilemmas" are simply functional dilemmas—problems that have evolved into dilemmas because they were not carefully considered. This is not a trivial point because unresolved problems can have the impact of a dilemma if problem solving is not successful.[50]

Unfortunately, most of the clinical ethics you have been taught has been about the 10 percent. Most ethical analysis in the clinical setting is not about the moral status of the fetus or the ethical propriety of physician-assisted suicide, embryonic stem cell research, or cloning. Rather it is about problems that can be addressed and resolved with careful attention to narrative details and clinical facts. In much the same way that the use of the GCAT can help prevent turning problems into dilemmas, a good ethics consult can help transform a brewing dilemma back into a problem with which you can work.

In addition to ethics consultation, ethics committees work to prevent the very cases they are consulted upon. They do this by engaging in educational outreach on cases and on the policies and procedures they are asked to draft. Typical issues include a large number that relate to patients at the end of life including brain death, medical futility, resuscitation, advance care planning, palliative care, and pain management.

You should try to involve yourself in the ethics consultation process should your patient require a consult and sit in all the meetings when it is appropriate. Each one of these cases can serve as a classroom in applied ethics. In addition, you might ask to attend a meeting of the hospital ethics committee and see how it operates and how such a diverse body achieves consensus judgments.

Signatures and Plans:

Print Names: MD/NP: _____

Nurse(s): _____

Social Worker: _____

Other(s): _____

Attending Assessment and Plan: _____

_____

Attending (print and sign): _____

Date: _____

Plans Reviewed with

Patient/Surrogate?   Yes [ ]   No [ ]   Date: _____

Specify: _____

Figure 10.4

The Centrality of Communication and Consensus

The accord that ethics committees try to achieve after disagreement emerges, is what goal setting can help achieve before conflict occurs. The final section of the GCAT seeks to document a level of accord between patient and/or family as well as the different members of the clinical team.

If that effort is successful, the process will culminate in a consensus amongst all those who are involved. A consensus is an agreement in opinion and is philologically linked to the voluntary agreement that characterizes *consent*. For our purposes, consensus represents agreement on the goals of care. This convergence of views is the exact opposite of the fractured dynamic, which marks a futility dispute where patient, families, and clinicians have divergent views about realizeable goals.

Although its completion can be taken as merely a bureaucratic notation in the medical record, it is symbolically the most critical section of the entire goal setting process. Here consensus is both a product, a decision that has been made about the goals of care, and the process itself, with process and decision both legitimating each other.[51]

Returning to this section of the GCAT, it signifies that all stakeholders are on the same page and that all who were entitled to be heard had the opportunity to voice an opinion and bring relevant information and perspectives to the table. It deliberately asks for the "sign-off" of the house officer or nurse practitioner directly providing care as well as that of the nurses and social worker involved in the patient's care. With this in place, it calls upon the attending physician to affirm the care plan and prompts the attending to review plans with the patient or surrogate. Each of these individuals, to one degree or another, is a stakeholder whose views have moral standing and deserve to be heard, if a legitimate consensus on the goals of care is to be reached.

It is especially important to include nurses and residents in this process because they provide the bulk of day-to-day care and because their voices may not be heard.[52,53] Though moral agents, each exists in a hierarchical relationship to their attending physicians when confronted by ethical issues at the end of life and can feel excluded and disenfranchised by and from the decision-making process.

Working with Nurses

Interdisciplinary collaboration with all members of the clinical team is essential for good end-of-life care, but working with your nursing colleagues is especially critical. It is important to include nurses and residents in this process because they provide the bulk of day-to-day care and because their voices may not be heard.[53] Although nurses may have more experience and clinical judgment than a novice physician, the organizational structure of care may lead to the marginalization of their input, often undermining interdisciplinary efforts so essential to good end-of-life care.

Strong collaboration leads to improved patient care and outcomes. One study of nurse–physician collaboration in the ICU indicates that nurse perceptions about the degree of collaboration were positively correlated with better patient outcomes.[54] Although this study did not specifically address palliative care, it did highlight the importance of nurse–physician collaboration in decisions regarding transfer of patients into and out of the ICU. Because we have viewed such nodal decision points as opportunities to readdress goals of care (See trigger 7), optimizing collaborative efforts with nursing is critical.

Think carefully about the quality of your collaborations with nursing colleagues. Although you might believe them adequate, an emerging literature on the sociology of the relationship between doctors and nurses suggests that nurses need a higher degree of collaboration to function successfully than their physician colleagues. Even when nurses and doctors objectively agree with the degree of collaboration, satisfaction levels differed.[55,56]

This caveat is more than a desire to have a harmonious team. Having the technical[57] and humanistic engagement[58] of your nursing colleagues in patient care brings the added skill sets of nursing and different modes of care to the bedside. One nurse commentator writing of the potential synergisms that are the fruits of collaboration has observed that, "the combination of nurses' style of decision making with that of physicians may enrich ethical decision making."[59]

Beyond questions of enrichment, though, is the basic issue of getting the job done and ensuring that adequate palliative care—and pain management—is provided. Simply put, this cannot happen if your nursing colleagues are estranged and do not feel part of the team and engaged in the decision-making process. I recall rounding in a medical intensive care unit shortly after David Asch published a paper on whether nurses believed that they had helped patients die in the ICU.[60] Although there was some confusion over definitional issues like double effect and the inappropriate use of opioids to intentionally hasten death (See Chapter 8 on the ethics of opioid use), a large number of nurses, 16 percent, reported that they thought they had helped patients die. This became the focus of our discussion.

I remember how these nurses were concerned about providing "too much" analgesic medication, lest anyone construe that they might be aiding in assisted suicide. One nurse said she would not give a large dose of medication, even if it were medically needed, because of the fear of sanction. She was categorical, and I remember precisely what she said: "Not on my license." By that she meant she was not going out on a limb. She was not going to assume unilateral responsibility for an action that could lead to disciplinary action, one that could even possibly jeopardize her nursing license.

We talked more about her stance. Other nurses agreed. They felt isolated from their physician colleagues over pain medication orders and had been "burned" in the past when they used a degree of clinical discretion and were not backed up by physicians. Instead of putting themselves in jeopardy, they had decided to treat pain conservatively and bear witness to patient suffering while imploring their physician colleagues to write more appropriate orders.

These nurses were unwilling to use their considerable clinical experience because they did not trust or feel comfortable with their physician colleagues, because they did not perceive a spirit of collaboration when a patient's orders authorized a range of dosing. They would not escalate the dose to the needed level but deliver medications in lower ranges so as not to be construed, in any way, of violating the law. Although these beliefs were in part a reflection of their knowledge regarding the ethics of opioid use, it also points to the sort of alienation that too often exists between physicians and their nursing colleagues who are charged with implementing doctors' orders.

Ensuring the cooperation of your colleagues in nursing is critical if you want to provide optimal palliative care to your patients. If the nurses do not agree with the plan of care, you are obliged to discuss it with them. In my experience, most disagreements between doctors and nurses occur when nurses are not in the loop, did not participate in the decision-making process, or were deprived of an essential bit of information about the patient's diagnosis or prognosis which may have lead to a rethinking of the goals of care.

The bottom line about working with nurses is simple. They are an indispensable part of the clinical team and must have a role in the decisions made for your mutual patients. Estranging them from this process is ill-advised, as you will count on them to deliver the bulk of care and need their counsel about your patient's needs and expectations. And because of their proximity to patients and families, nurses are well-positioned to support any consensus that might have emerged for palliation.

Involving the Patient and Family

This section also reminds us of the importance of communicating the plan of care with patient and family. Much of what we do clinically is behind-the-scenes work and not apparent to patients and families. It is critical to set up a family meeting, review plans, entertain questions, and allow for the process to work itself out. Families will need time to accommodate themselves to a decision to forgo curative care or to pursue palliation. Although the reasonableness of such an approach may seem obvious to you after reviewing the medical facts and considering the patient's preferences, patients and their families will likely want to hear it again, review the information, and work through the process, given the significance of their decision.

Although you might find such family meetings to be time-consuming, they are really essential to the health and well-being of the family unit. I recall a case involving a decision to withdraw life-sustaining measures from a patient with a poor prognosis following a coma. Although it was most likely the patient would remain in a minimally-conscious state,[61] there was a slim chance that there might be some hope for an additional level of recovery and possibly interaction with loved ones.[62]

It was clear from our knowledge of the patient's preferences that she would not want to live if there was no prospect of a life of the mind, which included the ability to read books and communicate in a meaningful way with family and loved ones. Meeting with the family allowed for a discussion of whether these goals, set by the patient while well in an advance directive, could be achieved or not. It allowed the goals to direct the care plan and provided solace to a family that decided to let go.

These meetings are never easy but they are indeed indispensable. Your presence bears witness and testifies to the importance of the meeting and the process of closure. Your engagement can help ensure that the process is thorough. More importantly, you can use such meetings to help heal families and prevent the fractures that can occur when tensions are high.

While none of these interventions can ease all the pain of loss, they can provide some support and prevent a complicated bereavement marked by second-guessing, recriminations, and normal melancholia turned to depression.[63]

One Good Death

Not all deaths can be good ones but most can be better. In closing, I would like to remember one that was better than expected and far better than most.

The patient was a gritty executive who had battled cancer for years. He had chosen to pursue aggressive therapies and participate in clinical trials and his life had been extended a number of times even beyond the most optimistic of projections. Throughout his course, he had been cared for by a wonderful attending physician with whom he had an excellent and frank relationship. They were indeed partners in their efforts to achieve his goal of prolonging life and avoiding unnecessary and avoidable pain and suffering.

Years earlier, when confronted by one challenging set of clinical circumstances after another, they had a conversation about what this old business man might want to do when his time was up and when available cures had finally eluded him. He told his attending he had always dreamt of writing poetry. He had always wanted to be a poet and when it was time, well, that's what he would do.

One morning on rounds we went to the patient's room with particularly bad news. All his new complaints, which had brought on a pain crisis, were the consequence of a grave recurrence of his disease. This patient, who had been so lucky, had finally had his luck run out.

We weren't quite sure what would be said at the bedside. After all, the man had been here before and had lived to tell the tale. He was a survivor and probably thinking that this time would be like the last and the one before that.

The attending sat at the bedside, adjusted a pillow, and looked him in the eyes. "I think it's time to write poetry," she said.

And he simply said, "Good."

References

1 *The Shorter Oxford English Dictionary on Historical Principles.* New York: Clarendon Press–Oxford University Press, 1987.

2 World Health Organization. *Cancer Pain Relief and Palliative Care.* Geneva, Switzerland: World Health Organization, 1990:11–12.

3 Spiess JL, Northcott CJ, Offsay JD, et al. Palliation Care: Something Else We Can Do for our Patients. *Psychiatric Service* 53(12)(2002): 1525–1529.

4 Kofkin, MI. Personal communication with author, 2004.

5 Roth, LH, Meisel A and Lidz CW. Tests of Competency to Consent to Treatment. *American Journal of Psychiatry* 134(3)(1977):279–284.

6 Zaubler TS, Viederman M, and Fins JJ. Ethical, Legal, and Psychiatric Issues in Capacity, Competence, and Informed Consent: An Annotated Bibliography. *General Hospital Psychiatry* 18(3)(1996):155–172.

7 Katz M, Abbey S, Rydall A, et al. Psychiatric Consultation for Competency to Refuse Medical Treatment: A Retrospective Study of Patient Characteristics and Outcome. *Psychosomatics* 36(1)(1995):33–41.

8 Trevor-Deutsch B and Nelson RF. Refusal of Treatment, Leading to Death: Towards Optimization of Informed Consent. *Annals Royal College of Physicians and Surgeons of Canada* 29(8)(1996):487–489.

9 Umapathy C, Ramchandani D, Lamdan RM, et al. Competency Evaluations on the Consultation–Liaison Service. Some Overt and Covert Aspects. *Psychosomatics* 40(1)(1999):28–33.

10 Leeman CP, Blum J and Lederberg MS. A Combined Ethics & Psychiatric Consultation. *General Hospital Psychiatry* 23(2)(2001):73–76.

11 Block SD. ACP-ASIM End-of-Life Care Consensus Panel. Assessing and Managing Depression in the Terminally Ill Patient. *Annals of Internal Medicine* 132(3)(2000):209–218.

12 Breitbart W and Strout D. Delirium in the Terminally Ill. *Clinics in Geriatric Medicine* 16(2)(2000):357–372.

13 Breitbart W, Bruera E, Chochinov H, et al. Neuropsychiatric Syndromes and Psychological Symptoms in Patients with Advanced Cancer. *Journal of Pain and Symptom Management* 10(2)(1995):131–141.

14 Adler LE and Griffith JM. Concurrent Medical Illness in the Schizophrenic Patient: Epidemiology, Diagnosis, and Management. *Schizophrenic Research* 4(2)(1991):91–107.

15 Breitbart W, Gibson C, Poppito SR, et al. Psychotherapeutic Interventions at the End of Life: A Focus on Meaning and Spirituality. *Canadian Journal of Psychiatry* 49(6)(2004):366–372.

16 Barnhill JW. "Psychotherapy of the Dying Patient" presented at Grand Rounds, Beth Israel Medical Center. New York, New York. March 25, 2004. (Personal copy of presentation to author)

17 Kunkel EJ, Woods CM, Rodgers C, et al. Consultations for 'Maladaptive Denial of Illness' Patients with Cancer: Psychiatric Disorders that Result in Noncompliance. *Psychooncology* 6(2)(1997):139–149.

18 Perry S and Viederman M. Management of Emotional Illness to Acute Medical Illness. *Medical Clinics of North America* 65(1)(1981):3–14.

19 Viederman M. The Pscyhodynamic Life Narrative: A Psychotherapeutic Intervention Useful in Crisis Situations. *Psychiatry* 46(3)(1983): 236–246.

20 Viederman M and Perry SW, 3rd. Use of Psychodynamic Life Narrative in the Treatment of Depression in the Physically Ill. *General Hospital Psychiatry* 2(3)(1980):177–185.

21 The Fetzer Institute. *Spiritual Beliefs and the Dying Process: A Report on a National Survey.* Princeton: The George H Gallup International Institute, 1997.

22 Hart CW. Spiritual Health, Illness, and Death. *Journal of Religion and Health* 33(1)(1994):17–22.

23 How to Meet JCAHO's Pastoral Care Standards. *Hospital Peer Review* 25(6)(2000):79–80.

24 Thiel MM and Robinson MR. Physicians' Collaboration with Chaplains: Difficulties and Benefits. *The Journal of Clinical Ethics* 8(1)1997):94–103.

25 Hart CW. Pastoral Care and Medical Education. *Journal of Religion and Health* 38(1)(1999):5–13.

26 I am grateful to Christine Cabochan-Manomat for locating New Testament verse for use here.

27 Drane JF. *More Humane Medicine: A Liberal Catholic Biotethics.* Edinboro, Pennsylvania: Edinboro University Press, 2003.

28 Catholic Health Association. Care of the Dying: A Catholic Perspective. Part III: Clinical Context—Good Palliative Care Eases the Dying Process. *Health Progress* 74(4)(1993):22–26, 31.

29 Ehman JW, Ott BB, Short TH, et. al. Do Patients Want Physicians to Inquire About Their Spiritual or Religious Beliefs If They Become Gravely Ill? *Archives of Internal Medicine* 159(15)(1999):1803–1806.

30 Post SG, Puchalski CM and Larson DB. Physician and Patient Spirituality: Professional Boundaries, Competency and Ethics. *Annals of Internal Medicine* 132(7)(2000):578–583.

31 Lo B, Ruston D, Kates LW et al. Discussing Religious and Spiritual Issues at the End of Life: A Practical Guide for Physicians. *Journal of the American Medical Association* 287(6)(2002):749–754.

32 Puchalski C. Spirituality in Health: The Role of Spirituality in Critical Care. *Critical Care Clinics* 20(3)(2004):487–504.

33 Lo B, Kates LW, Ruston D et al. Responding to Requests Regarding Prayer and Religious Ceremonies by Patients Near the End of Life and their Families. *Journal of Palliative Medicine* 6(3)(2003):409–415.

34 Fins JJ, Peres JR, Schumacher JD and Meier C. *On the Road from Theory to Practice: A Resource Guide to Promising Practices in Palliative Care Near the End of Life.* Washington, DC: Last Acts National Program Office, Robert Wood Johnson Foundation, 2003.

35 National Consensus Project for Quality Palliative Care. *Clinical Practice Guidelines for Quality Palliative Care.* May 2004.

36 Campbell ML and Frank RR. Experience with an End-of-life Practice at a University Hospital. *Critical Care Medicine* 25(1)(1997):197–202.

37 Fins JJ, Gentilesco BJ, Carver A, et al. Reflective Practice and Palliative Care Education: A Clerkship Responds to the Informal and Hidden Curriculum. *Academic Medicine* 78(3)(2003):307–312.

38 Poretnoy R. Personal communication to author, 2004.

39 Foster LW and McLellan LJ. Translating Psychosocial Insight into Ethical Discussions Supportive of Patients in End-of-life Decisionmaking. *Social Work in Health Care* 35(2)(2002):37–51.

40 Hogan C, Luney J, Gabel J, et al. Medicare Beneficiaries' Cost of Care in the Last Year of Life. *Health Affairs* 20(4)(2001):188–195.

41 This section draws in part from: Agrawal SK and Fins JJ. Ethics Committees and Case Consultation in the Hospital Setting. *A Guide to Hospitals and Inpatient Care.* Siegler E, Mirafzali S, and Foust JB, (Eds.) New York: Springer, 2003.

42 Fletcher JC and Siegler M. What Are the Goals of Ethics Consultation? *Journal of Clinical Ethics* 7(2)(1996):122–126.

43 Wolf SM. Ethics Committees and Due Process: Nesting Rights in a Community of Caring. *Maryland Law Review* 50(3)(1991):798–858.

44 Leeman CP, Fletcher JC, Spencer EM, et al. Quality Control For Hospitals' Clinical Ethics Services: Proposed Standards. *Cambridge Quarterly of Healthcare Ethics* 6(3)(1997):257–268.

45 Fletcher JC and Hoffmann DE. Ethics Committees: Time to Experiment with Standards. *Annals of Internal Medicine* 120(4)(1994):335–338.

46 SHHV-SBC Task Force on Standards for Bioethics Consultation. *Core Competencies for Health Care Ethics Consultation,* 1998.

47 Dubler N and Nimmons D. *Ethics on Call.* New York: Harmony Books, 1992.

48 Fetters MD, Churchill L, and Danis M. Conflict Resolution at the End of Life. *Critical Care Medicine* 29(5)(2001):1078–1079.
49 I am indebted to my colleague Franklin G. Miller for the helpful distinction between a dilemma and a problem.
50 Fins JJ, Bacchetta MD and Miller FG. Clinical Pragmatism: A Method of Moral Problem Solving. *Kennedy Institute of Ethics* 7(2)(1997):129–145.
51 Moreno JD. *Deciding Together.* New York: Oxford University Press, 1995.
52 Fins JJ and Nilson EG. An Approach to Educating Residents about Palliative Care and Clinical Ethics. *Academic Medicine* 75(6)(2000):662–665.
53 Solomon MZ, O'Donnell L, Jennings B, et al. Decisions Near the End of Life: Professional Views on Life-Sustaining Treatments. *American Journal of Public Health* 83(1)(1993):14–23.
54 Baggs JG, Schmitt MH, Mushlin AI, et al. Association Between Nurse–Physician Collaboration and Patient Outcomes in Three Intensive Care Units. *Critical Care Medicine* 27(9)(1999):1991–1998.
55 Baggs JD, Schmitt MH, Mushlin AI, et al. Nurse–Physician Collaboration and Satisfaction with the Decision-Making Process in Three Critical Care Units. *American Journal of Critical Care* 6(5)(1997):393–399.
56 Baggs JD and Schmitt MH. Intensive Care Decisions about Levels of Aggressiveness of Care. *Research in Nursing & Health* 18(4)(1995):345–355.
57 Ferrell BR and Coyle N. An Overview of Palliative Care Nursing. *American Journal of Nursing* 102(5)(2002):26–31.
58 Baggs JD. Collaborative Interdisciplinary Bioethical Decision Making in Intensive Care Units. *Nursing Outlook* 41(3)(1993):108–112.
59 Ibid, p. 109.
60 Asch DA. The Role of Critical Care Nurses in Euthanasia and Assisted Suicide. *New England Journal of Medicine* 334(21)(1996):1374–1379.
61 Giacino JT, Ashwal S, Childs N, et al. The Minimally Conscious State: Definition and Diagnostic Criteria. *Neurology* 58(3)(2002):349–353.
62 Fins JJ. Rethinking Disorders of Consciousness: New Research and Its Implications. *Hastings Center Report* 35(2)(2005):22–24.
63 Holland JC. Management of Grief and Loss: Medicine's Obligation and Challenge. *Journal of the American Medical Women's Association* 57(2)(2002):95–96.

A p p e n d i x

The Goals of Care Assessment Tool

Triggers Completion of GCAT

Terminal Status Perceived

1. Clinician Perceptions: [ ]
   - Clinician(s) consider that the patient may be dying.
2. Patient or Surrogate Perceptions: [ ]
   - Patient indicates an awareness/concern that s/he may be dying or wish to die.
   - Surrogate indicates awareness/concern that patient is dying or expresses hope that patient will die soon.
   - Patient or surrogate expresses preference for comfort care, palliative care, or hospice.

End-of-Life Decisions

3. Clinicians consider/recommend end-of-life care options: [ ]
   - Advance care planning
   - Withholding of life-sustaining therapy (e.g., DNR order)
   - Withdrawal of life-sustaining therapy
   - Hospice or palliative care referral
4. Patient/Surrogate considers or agrees to end-of-life care options: [ ]
   - Advance care planning
   - Withholding of life-sustaining therapy (e,g., DNR order)
   - Withdrawal of life-sustaining therapy
   - Hospice or palliative care referral

Medical Developments

5. New Diagnostic or Prognostic Information: [ ]
   - Diagnosis of life-threatening illness.
   - Prognosis of < 6months life expectancy.
6. Change in Clinical Course in Patient With Life-Threatening Illness: [ ]
   - Acute decompensation: e.g., respiratory failure, sepsis, shock, significant change in mental status.
   - Need for life-sustaining therapy: e.g., pressors, ventilator, tube feeding, dialysis.
7. Admission/Transfer to ICU: [ ]
   - Goals should be reassessed upon consideration of ICU Admission.
8. Refractory End-of-Life Symptoms: [ ]
   - Unrelieved distress from pain, dyspnea, anxiety, depression, nausea/vomiting, or constipation.

Clinical Assessment

To Be Completed by Primary Care-Giver (House Officer, Nurse Practitioner, Or Attending Physician)

Name: _____ Age: _____
Hospital # _____
Today's Date: _____ Date of Admission: _____
Floor: _____ Service: _____ Attending: _____
Diagnosis: _____

Assessment of Capacity and the Refusal of Life-Sustaining Therapies

Patient Capacity: Comments:
Yes [ ]   Variable [ ]   _____
No [ ]   Unclear [ ]   _____

Knowledge of Diagnosis and Prognosis

Information:

	Yes	No	Unknown	Comments:
Patient aware of diagnosis	[ ]	[ ]	[ ]	_____
Patient aware of prognosis	[ ]	[ ]	[ ]	_____
Friend/Family/Surrogate aware of diagnosis	[ ]	[ ]	[ ]	_____
aware of prognosis	[ ]	[ ]	[ ]	_____

Articulated Preferences for End-of-Life Care

Preferences Regarding Life-Sustaining Therapy:

	Yes	No	Unknown
DNR	[ ]	[ ]	[ ]

Comments: _____

	Yes	No	Unknown
Advance Directive	[ ]	[ ]	[ ]

_____

	Yes	No	Unknown
Health Care Proxy:	[ ]	[ ]	[ ]

_____

	Yes	No	Unknown
Living Will:	[ ]	[ ]	[ ]

_____

Name: _____
Phone: _____

Placing the Patient in Context

Family Support:

	Yes	No	Unknown
Does patient have friends/family	[ ]	[ ]	[ ]
Involved Family	[ ]	[ ]	[ ]

  Identified Spokesperson(s): _____
  Relationship: _____
  Family preferences: _____
Psychosocial issues: _____
Cultural issues: _____
Discussion with Patient/Family: _____

Pain and Symptom Inventory

Symptom:	Yes	No	Treated/Response:
Pain	[ ]	[ ]	_____
Anxiety	[ ]	[ ]	_____
Depression	[ ]	[ ]	_____
Cognitive Dysfunction	[ ]	[ ]	_____
Dyspnea	[ ]	[ ]	_____
Diarrhea	[ ]	[ ]	_____
Nausea/Vomiting	[ ]	[ ]	_____
Constipation	[ ]	[ ]	_____
Other Suffering	[ ]	[ ]	_____

Specify: _____

Goals of Care

Cure	[ ]
Restore Function	[ ]
Prolong Life	[ ]
Comfort Care/Palliation	[ ]

Comments: _____
_____

Planned Interventions   Comments:

Psychiatry Consult [ ]   _____

Pastoral Care Visit [ ]   _____

Pain Service/Palliative Care Consult [ ]   _____

Referral to Palliative Care Unit [ ]   _____

Hospice Referral [ ]   _____

Social Work [ ]   _____

Ethics Committee [ ]   _____

Other [ ]   _____

Consensus

Signatures and Plans:

Print Names: MD/NP: _____   Nurse(s): _____

Social Worker: _____   Other(s): _____

Attending Assessment and Plan: _____
_____

Attending (print and sign): _____ Date: _____

Plans Reviewed with Patient/Surrogate?   Yes [ ]   No [ ]

Date: _____

Specify: _____

Index

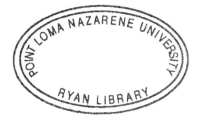